THE

VIOLET RAY

BOOK

INCLUDING

EDGAR CAYCE READINGS

AND

OLD MANUSCRIPTS

This book is for Research and Educational Purposes Only.
Information printed does not constitute advice. Information printed in this booklet is not intended to medically prescribe or promote the sale of any product, nor is it intended to replace qualified medical care.

IMPORTANT NOTE: This book is compiled for those that are interested in the Violet Ray. Nothing in this book is to be considered as medical advice. If you have a medical condition, contact a qualified health care professional. None of the information or ideas in this book are a substitute for the advice of a licensed physician.

FOREWORD

During the early 1900's, Violet Ray instructional booklets were included with the purchase of a Violet Ray machine. The chapters titled *How to Treat with Violet Rays, The Scientific Method of Combating Pain,* The Halliwell Shelton High Frequency Violet Ray Manual *For Beauty and Better Health* and the RenuLife Electric Company *Violet Ray For Health, Strength, Beauty* are all examples of those booklets. For those researching the history and application of these machines, this information is both informative and insightful as to the type of therapies used during this time.

In addition to examples of the booklets provided, we have also included excerpts from the Edgar Cayce Health Care Philosophy. These excerpts reference suggested applications of this machine given by Cayce during the period of time that he provided "readings" to individuals requesting his assistance. We have attempted to balance the claims of early manufacturers of this Violet Ray machine with the usefulness of the machine as presented in the Edgar Cayce readings.

During the early 1900's, electrotherapy and light therapy were used quite often and were considered standard medical practice. With the introduction of antibiotics and other drug discoveries, this science took a back seat. Today, there is a resurgence of interest in electrotherapy and light therapy.

Bruce Baar MS, ND

For further information, please contact:

Baar Products, Inc.
Post Office Box 60
Downingtown, PA 19335
610-873-4591
www.baar.com

TABLE OF CONTENTS

This is an excerpt from an old Violet Ray instructional book that was available during the early 1900's and was supplied with the Violet Ray's that were available at that time. Note that many of the claims for the Violet Ray provided in this section have not yet been supported by medical documentation.

How To Treat with Violet Rays
author unknown

ONE CAUSE FOR ALL DISEASE AND WEAKNESS

All human ailments, with the exception of highly infectious and contagious diseases, are traceable to one cause: Imperfect circulation and impoverished blood.

During our youth, when we take plenty of exercise, enjoy sound sleep, our blood is rich and we are insured of a copious supply to every part of our body.

Gradually, as we grow older, we pursue a more sedate mode of living and our circulation slows down at the same time. The flow of blood through our veins is slower and our whole body suffers.

When our body is in this condition, germs find fertile field to lodge and multiply.

For this reason, weak and run-down persons become easy prey to almost any disease to which they are exposed.

How To Remedy This Condition

It is reasonable to assume that by increasing the flow of blood through the body, the reverse of this process will be true and the congestion and disorder can be relieved.

A systematic course in physical culture will, in time, renovate the body completely. Few of us are able to devote necessary time to such course. By means of Violet Ray treatment, every functional activity of the body can be sped up and the blood made to run through the veins with renewed vigor.

Concentration

An important feature of this treatment is that it can be concentrated to any particular organ that requires special treatment. It brings a vigorous surge of rich warm blood to any part, thereby washing away the silt of disease, strengthening and nourishing the tissues, and giving vigor and vitality to any part treated.

What The Violet Ray Is

The Violet Ray High Frequency Current, or as it is more commonly called, the "Violet Ray", is a new phase of electricity. It is applied to any part of the human body without pain, muscular contraction or disagreeable sensation of any kind. The electrical oscillations representing the High Frequency Current follow each other with such tremendous rapidity that they outspeed our nervous sensibility; we do not become conscious of their presence: in other words our nerves are insensitive to the electrical oscillations of the Violet Ray. The oscillations are so rapid that they exceed many thousand repetitions per second. The Violet Rays are pleasing, and though most stimulating and highly invigorating to the entire system, nerves, and muscles, cannot record the presence of their great power.

What Violet Rays Accomplish

Violet Rays or High Frequency Currents benefit all living matter. Through the glass vacuum applicator light, heat, electric energy and ozone are created. These forces are uniformly potent in relieving and eliminating human ailments. Violet Rays present a remedy upon which we can rely. They are positive and certain in action. They will reach where medicine does not, and often cannot — yet they cause no pain, no disagreeable sensation or discomfort. They furnish a soothing relief. They destroy germs and have a strong power over infection.

A Violet Ray treatment is the surest method of relieving pain. Applied to that part of the body where the pain is severest, the rays and High Frequency electrical discharge penetrate every cell, tissue and organ and tranquilize and soothe. They build up the forces of nutrition and general health. Violet Rays will stimulate and strengthen the vital organs, develop the body and steady the nerves, spraying thousands of volts of High-Frequency electricity into any weak, sluggish or painful organ or muscle, purifying and causing the flow of warm rich blood to surge through the treated part, at the same time being painless and pleasant. Violet Rays have only to be tried to be appreciated.

Cellular Message

Every vibration of the Violet Ray causes the cells of the body to vibrate. This vibration gives the effect of massage, and as its frequency is so high that it is insensible to us, its effect is rapid and powerful.

It imparts new life to each individual cell and enables it to more readily absorb the nutriment from the blood stream, thereby building new tissue. In short, it tends to revive and invigorate every bodily tissue by rejuvenating each individual cell of which it is composed.

Summary Effect of Violet Ray Treatment

When Daily treatments are given with Violet Rays the following effects are observed:

- Return of sleep
- Increase of strength and vital energy
- Increase in cheerfulness and power for work
- Improvement in appetite, digestion, etc.
- Increase of blood supply to the point of application
- General increase of local nutrition and progressive improvement in the general functions
- Increase of secretions
- Increase of oxygen in the blood. (Ozone being driven directly through the skin into the tissues, accomplishing "ozonization" of the blood)

Why You Should Use Violet Rays

Violet Rays should be used by everyone experiencing sickness or ailment of any kind. The healing properties of Violet Rays are manifold, and they accomplish what drugs and medicine never can. The regular introduction of a vitalizing shower of diffused electricity into your system is exactly what is needed to make it function properly and efficiently. To be healthy, use Violet Rays.

There are three distinctly different ways of applying the Violet Ray:

First: Soothing Effect.
This soothing or sedative effect is administered by means of the glass applicator. To secure this effect, the applicator is applied directly to the bare skin. You can calm painful sensation by sedative treatment: these treatments are of great benefit to all nervous ailment. Nervous troubles are quickly and most beneficially influenced by the sedative currents. A general electrification treatment refreshes the entire nervous system.

Second: Stimulating Tonic and Invigoration.
Stimulation and invigoration are produced whenever an electrode is somewhat lifted during its application or used through cloth or clothing.

This stimulation is caused by the many small sparks called the High Frequency Spray. They bombard the area which they cover, causing a tingling but pleasant sensation. They have a beneficial heating effect, too. Besides they generate ozone. Particles of this ozone are driven right into the tissues, causing ozonization of the blood. Sparks are also germ-killing and have a great power over infection.

Stimulating treatments are best produced by application through the clothing or through a towel which has been put over the part to be treated. As the length of the stimulating spray depends on the thickness of the interposed dry resistance, that is the clothing or towel, any desired effect is obtainable. Anything from a handkerchief to a doubled Turkish towel can be used for this purpose. The use of any kind of cloth insures a uniformity in spark length which cannot be obtained in any other way. Powdering the skin with talcum powder often suffices to create the desired dry resistance. This will, at the same time, allow an easy sliding of the applicator. A slight perspiration results from the treatment-this is natural. If the application of talcum powder is not desirable, use of lubricant is recommended.

Stimulating treatment through clothing finds a profound use in rheumatism, lumbago, partial paralysis, etc. Slight stimulation is also sometimes desired in skin troubles where the blood circulation is impaired. A single layer of handkerchief presents enough resistance in such a case. Chronic rheumatic troubles, however, may require the use of several layers or a Turkish towel.

Long sparks from the applicator will cause counter irritation. Counter irritation quickly relieves pains of many sorts.

It is often the very welcome means to kill the pain of a toothache. You will appreciate this pain-relieving quality of the Violet Ray also in sprains, strains, bruises, etc. Counter irritating applications are better, swifter and more effective than plasters and liniments. In fact, they replace them entirely. Stimulating treatments are long lasting in their effects. They are not like drugs or a glass of wine because they are not followed by a reaction. They do not create any habits.

Third: Internal Antiseptic.
The effect of inhaling ozone is much the same as that of inhaling copious quantities of pure air. It purifies and enriches the blood, invigorates the body, and causes pure oxygen to be taken up in large quantities in the blood stream.

Ozone inhalation is of particular benefit in the treatment of respiratory disorders. Taken into the lungs, it immediately attacks the disease cells and causes them to be oxidized and thrown off with the exhaled air. This treatment has been found to be of great benefit in cases of bronchitis, colds on the lungs, tuberculosis and similar troubles.
(Author's Note: Excess amounts of ozone in the lungs can be damaging.)

Pain Relieving

Rheumatism
The blood deposits poisons when the circulation becomes sluggish, usually at the joints and we feel a slight pain. Continued deposits cause the joints to swell and inflammation to set in. This is called articular rheumatism. The same condition causes pain in the muscles and we have muscular rheumatism.

Violet Rays restore circulation and drive oxygen into the blood, thereby, bringing back to a normal condition the afflicted part.

The Condensor Electrode is found most beneficial and should be taken twice daily with a medium strength current. The very first treatment brings a warm, glowing tinge to the skin and relief is apparent.

Neuritis
This may be treated in a similar manner as rheumatism, only with a milder current.

Lumbago

This is treated like rheumatism, preferably through the clothing, and with a strong current and with the condensor electrode, twice a day.

Headaches-Insomnia-Brain Fag

When the blood collects in pools throughout the body, it becomes stagnant. One of the most troublesome of these is the cavity in the skull where it directly affects the brain. This causes headaches, brain fag, and insomnia. Everyone knows that prolonged mental effort will bring about a congestion in the brain that dulls our power of thought. When this is demanded over a long period of time, circulation is impaired, the nerves irritated and the familiar, dull headache, results. The general treatment is to use the surface electrode and apply it to the different parts of the head, thereby relieving the congestion.

Hair-Scalp-Skin

The hair roots are fed, just as every other part of the body is, through the blood. For treatment of the scalp we have a special comb applicator which pulls easily through the hair and conforms to the shape of the head. Millions of tiny electric sparks carry pure ozone to the capillaries through which the blood flows in the scalp. These tiny capillaries are gently massaged, and nourishment is brought to the roots of the hair. The very first treatment brings a long, glowing, healthy feeling to the scalp, and with few successive treatments, itching will stop, hair will cease falling, and dandruff disappear. In many cases, gray hair will even be restored to its natural color. By stimulating the scalp apparently dead hair will quickly take on a natural glossy and healthy appearance.

The Violet Ray applied to the face, brings fresh, rich oxygen-laden blood, which cleanses the pores, dissolves poisons and other waste matter and assists nature to produce a natural, glowing, healthy condition or complexion. One short treatment every evening and every morning will work wonders on the complexion.

Run Down-Condition

General weakness, tiredness, loss of weight, lack of appetite, indicate anemia or impoverished blood and poor circulation. The Violet Ray stands alone as the most potent treatment known to science in giving quick relief to such disorders.

This treatment is taken with the general body applicator over the entire body for five minutes, twice daily, using a medium current. The metal applicator is also very beneficial and should be held firmly in the hands for ten minutes, twice daily, with a strong current which massages the body with a stimulating cellular massage. Ozone inhalations give very beneficial results.

Dyspepsia, Constipation and Digestive Disorders

This treatment consists in getting the blood into circulation so that it will find its way to the lungs to be properly purified. Then the digestive organs must be stimulated to function properly, so they will rid themselves of the accumulation of bodily waste. Its great advantage over medical treatment is that it can be applied directly to the seat of trouble.

For the relief of indigestion and constipation, the current should be first applied to the abdomen. The applicator should be held in loose contact with the skin, so that a mildly stimulating effect is obtained. This, in turn, will speed up circulation, stimulate the muscles of the abdominal wall and relieve the congested organs. Treatment of the spinal nerve centers should follow the above treatment.

11

Strengthening the Reproductive System

The various weaknesses that afflict these organs in both men and women spring from the same general causes as most other bodily weaknesses, and must be treated accordingly.

Correcting Female Complaints

It is true that the sexual system, particularly in women, is very delicately adjusted, and, consequently, any disorder affecting other parts of the body may have an influence on this system. Women suffering from anemia, obesity, digestive disturbances and nervous disorders will, in nine cases out of ten, suffer from female troubles also. Because of this, they usually resort to treatment with some nostrum that acts directly on the organs instead of getting at the fundamental cause of the trouble.

In women, disorders of this kind may be classified into three groups: The first group includes those caused by weakness of the parts or of the supporting ligaments and tissues. The second group includes nervous complaints and the third those resulting from internal infections. Into the first class may be placed all displacements and similar troubles that are so common and distressing. The second, or nervous disorders, may be regarded as functional disorders that contribute to the development of the first group. The third includes inflammations of all kinds in the pelvic region and manifest themselves through the several organs. Usually the symptoms indicate a complication of disorders falling into at least two of these classes.

Violet Ray treatment gives the most gratifying results in correcting disorders of this kind, for the reason that by proper application and treatment, the effects are both constitutional and local, which insures rapid improvement.

The third class of troubles mentioned-those caused by internal infections-are usually characterized by inflammation, pain, and frequently by unnatural discharges. The treatment described in the preceding paragraph should be used, and in addition internal treatment with one of the vaginal electrodes, preferably the insulating electrode. This internal application acts not only as a local antiseptic, but relieves inflammation as well. Applicators for administering internal treatment will be found in the back of this booklet. The duration of this should not exceed five or six minutes.

Author's note: Applicators for internal use are not currently available.

Treatment for Men

With men, disorders of the reproductive organs seldom cause the physical distress as with women, but their influence on the mental condition of the man is frequently even more severe. Men become afflicted with these troubles largely through the same causes as women — lack of exercise, faulty nutrition, nervous conditions, etc. These are all too frequently aggravated by excessive use of tobacco, alcohol and sexual indiscretions.

The same general tonic treatment prescribed for women should be taken by men also. In addition to this, great benefit will be derived from daily treatment of the external organs lasting for from five to seven minutes. This should be given with a medium current, keeping the applicator in loose contact with the skin so that a stimulating tonic effect is obtained.

Prostatic Troubles

Prostatic trouble becomes apparent in nearly all men after they reach the age of thirty-five or forty. The prostate gland is a small gland completely surrounding the urethra at the mouth of the bladder. Poor circulation, faulty nutrition, etc., cause this gland to become inflamed and swollen, and pain and agony results.

For permanent, lasting results, no other treatment will give the practically certain relief that comes from the use of the Violet Rays. Prominent physicians report the most beneficial results in nine out of ten cases.

Treatment should be taken with either our special prostatic or insulated rectal applicators. By means of this, heat is brought in almost direct contact with the gland inside the body and relief is experienced at once. The circulation is improved, nutriment and oxygen are brought directly to the gland and the inflammation and pain disappears as if by magic.

External treatment should be taken over the entire lower spine. This stimulates and builds up the network of nerves running to and around the gland. A mild current should be used for about five minutes daily.

Author's note: Applicators for internal use are not currently available.

IMPORTANT

ALWAYS unplug the Violet Ray from the electrical outlet. The adjustment knob on the instrument is to regulate the strength of current - **not to use as an on and off switch.**

NEVER use the generator when in a bathtub or when connection is made from the body to the ground, by radiators, water pipes, lighting fixtures, etc.

NEVER use generator on the hair when using at the same time a hair tonic containing a large percentage of alcohol.

NEVER oil the generator.

NEVER attempt to repair the generators.

Note: The Violet Ray Hand Machine cannot be used for more than 10 minutes at a time as the unit must then cool down.

CHAPTER II

Edgar Cayce Readings on the Violet Ray

*Note: The following excerpts from the Edgar Cayce readings do not include the reading in its entirety. For the complete reading, you may request it by referring to the reading number listed at the end of the excerpt.

EFFECTS OF THE VIOLET RAY

26. We would give, too, those vibrations from the *Violet Ray* anode that charges the body direct while being held in the hand. The anode would be held in the hand for five to eight minutes two or three times each week.

27. This treatment is to so charge the centers of the nervous system as to make for (with the changes created in the activities of that assimilated, in its distribution through the system) better coordination BETWEEN the sympathetic and cerebro-spinal nervous system. It would produce stimuli to the GANGLIA in the cerebro-spinal and sympathetic coordinating centers. 259-7/Nervous System: Incoordination/

****

24. ...we would begin with the *Violet Ray* treatments taken every other evening before retiring directly on the spine; this to stimulate the superficial circulation, especially, and revitalize, giving more activity to the whole of the respiratory system. The treatments should be for at least fifteen to twenty minutes. 388-1 /Circulation, Incoordination/

****

21. (Q) How long at a time should the *Violet Ray* be used?
(A) On the body itself from two to five minutes on either side; that is, ten minutes then in all - see? and burned, so that the air may be purified (that is, inhaled), for fifteen to twenty minutes; this not touching the body, of course, at all, but filling the room - or about the body - as well as possible, see? Under the existent conditions, of course, it's well for as much oxygen as possible. Hence the manner in which it has been kept about the body; but let these inhalations that come from burning about the body be so that they may be inhaled by the body. Not necessary to smother the body, of course, with sheets or covers - but burned in the room, so that it is ladened - or the fumes from same wafted over the body, see? 374-1 /Cancer, Lungs/

****

3. We would have each day the *Violet Ray* treatment, along the spine and over the throat where there are those tendencies for the non-activity of the glands from the thyroids and those accumulations and the fullness that appears in the throat. These will naturally be somewhat irritated at times by the electrical vibrations, but with the taking of properties for the glands themselves the body will gradually adjust itself. We would use the bulb applicator along the throat, up to the head, down the cerebrospinal system, for at least three to five minutes. THEN we would hold in the hand the application where the body charges, is charged by the electrical forces passing through same, for about five minutes. Do this each day, preferably before retiring at night. These will make for better conditions and ELECTRIFY, as it were, the energies of the system. 421-10 /Goiter: Tendencies/

****

25. (Q) What causes pain in mornings through my back and stomach?
(A) As indicated, this is that particular area where there should be the applications of the *Violet Ray* for the superficial activity, as well as the effectiveness that this will be through the corrective measures in the solar plexus area as indicated. The cause, then, is from incoordination in the sympathetic and cerebro-spinal, in the solar plexus area; making for the hypogastric contraction that produces the stomach disturbances. And naturally, with same comes the effective forces across the small of the back, in the form of pain produced by contraction of the muscular forces, by incoordination of the nerve plexus or ganglia itself. 268-2 /Spine: Subluxations/

****

7. Since all portions of the body aid or retard the conditions that have been involved, in a greater or lesser degree, and inasmuch as the general condition that first affected the body (catarrhal condition) has to do with the general circulation, we would find that an ASSISTANT to the circulation and lymph supply - as we have given - would be well; through the use occasionally - every two or three days, if not every day - of the *Violet Ray*, especially over the upper dorsal and cervical area. Not over head or ear at this time, but over those portions of system where the impulses from the nerve forces are to supply energy and circulation to the system - or to those portions that have been affected. 269-4/Ears, Deafness/

****

9. (Q) Should the light rays be given?
(A) Very good that the light rays be given, for this assists the blood in producing an equilibrium. 325-9 /Circulation, Incoordination/

****

10. ...only using the plain hand *Violet Ray* immediately or thirty minutes after the Ash has been taken into the system (and this may be taken, of course, at home - the plain Violet Ray, see?), using it over those portions of the body from the central dorsal system to the end of the toes, and particularly over those portions where the erosions or the conditions are to be centralized from the activity of the circulation in body. This then would only be taken once a week, see? 275-34 /Perth's Disease/

****

10. Preferably as the body is prepared for the evening rest, take one-eighth grain of the carbon ash - emptied from the capsule onto the tongue tend swallowed down with water -each evening.

11. Thirty minutes after the ash has been taken, apply the *violet ray* over the area of the upper dorsal and lower cervical area, for fifteen to thirty minutes with the bulb applicator; from the 9th dorsal to the 3rd or 4th cervical area; this whole area being covered at each treatment each evening, see?

12. This would make for the adding or releasing for the system the absorbed effects of the ash (that is, the *Violet Ray* treatment), such as to carry to the system more of oxygen in such a manner as to stimulate the resuscitating influences of a better equalized circulation, through the administration; and bring about, in a period of sixteen to twenty-eight days, a reaction that we find would be much more satisfactory. 407-1 /Neurasthenia/

****

6. In the presenting, or in the delivery, there was an injury primarily to the lower lumbar and sacral areas.

7. While this has prevented a normal development, naturally being to the nerve forces of the sensory or sympathetic system it has kept all the coordination between cerebrospinal and sympathetic from nominal development of the muscular and locomotory activity; through not an atrophy but an impaired development of the nerve tensions and the nerve connections through the ganglia in those areas as indicated.

8. These then as we find cause the weakened condition, the inclination for the body to easily become acid through its activities; and weakening the ability for resistance, or lacking in same, we find the general weakness occurs.

9. As we find, those administrations which have been made neuropathically are most excellent; but we would add this as the rub externally, - an equal combination of Peanut Oil and Olive Oil. The occasional use of the Cod Liver Oil is very well, but this taken internally will be found much preferable for the body, especially in the form of Cod Liver Oil and iron and the vitamins - as may be found in that called Codiron; this taken about one pellet twice each day, with the meal.

10. Also we would use the low electrical forces as from the very low form of electricity but in the high vibratory force, as found in the *Violet Ray* (hand machine, bulb applicator). This would be applied direct to the body, not too much at a time, and especially along the cerebrospinal system, and particularly in the area of the muscular force and the nerve tensions for arms and limbs, or the upper dorsal and cervical and the lumbar and the sacral and down the lower limbs. This will aid in their development, and as it were the "taking" of the activity of the manipulations, as well as absorptions through the oil rubs.

11. When this is first begun (the *Violet Ray*), do not give this more than a minute - over the whole body.

12. These should be kept almost every day; that is, the massage as well as the *Violet Ray*. 1805 /Birth Injuries, After Effects/

****

1. EC: We have the body here, [5456] - this we have had before. In many respects we find conditions improved. In some respects we find some irritations at times, which apparently is rather disconcerting, or discouraging to the body. These, we find, will be materially aided will there be the application of the *Violet Ray*, especially across the lumbar and sacral regions, following - or during the treatments, or the administering of the manipulation, or the general osteopathic adjustment AND manipulation.

These will aid materially in creating the better association of the rejuvenations as are being exercised in the system. These conditions, as we find, arise from what may be properly termed the reactions as come from the rejuvenating, or the re-exercising of nerve and muscular tissue as has been rather dormant. 5456-2 /Spine, Subluxations/

******

2. The conditions in the blood supply, produced by irritations that come from conditions in the cerebrospinal system, which - with their reactions upon the nervous system - produce those conditions in digestive system, in lungs, bronchi and throat, the seat or the cause - as we find - from irritations in the pelvic organs, or system, and make for a general irritation in the organs, producing improper functioning in same, with discharges that are IRRITATING to the body and produce a general nervous debilitation that gives more of the irritating to the rest of the functioning system.
3. Then, to meet or to overcome these conditions, there should be first the general attitude as to life, as to the spiritual environments of the body-consciousness, as to a faith, a trust, IN something.
4. There should be those manipulations and corrections in the cerebro-spinal system, that will alleviate the pressures in the lumbar and dorsal region, as well as alignments in the upper dorsal and cervical. These should be taken, as we would find, at least three to four times each week. These may be given either osteopathically or chiropractically, so that the ADJUSTMENTS or the alleviations are made.
5. Then, after each treatment, there should be the vibrations from the *Violet Ray* for at least three to four, to five minutes, over the WHOLE of the cerebrospinal system, to enliven the circulation OVER the centers that especially are adjusted. 5493/Leukorrhea/

******

17. We would first begin with the applications of a low form of electrical vibration that may be had through the use of the plain *Violet Ray*. Not the deep therapy, but the hand *violet ray* machine - which will act upon the superficial circulatory forces of the body - applied along the cerebrospinal system. This will relax the body and stimulate the ganglia along the whole cerebrospinal system. Use the plain bulb applicator each day, preferably as the body is ready for retirement, for a least five minutes. Move the bulb applicator rather in a circular motion from the center of the spine toward both extremities; that is, begin in the center and move upward - then begin in the center and move downward - but in a circular motion on each side of the spine from the brachial center, and also from the lumbar center. 931-2 /Eliminations/

******

12. For those conditions or abrasions in the skin, on the face and over the body - or portions of body - we would use the Violet Ray, STIMULATING - see - with the *Violet Ray* - those centers in the cerebrospinal system from which the PORTIONS in the skin, or face, or hands, or arms, or body (as it is), are active from the cerebrospinal system; that is, as for face, in the 1st and 2nd DORSAL and in the whole of the cervical area; not so much on those portions where abrasions show themselves. Do that. 947-1/Eliminations: Eczema/

******

OZONE EFFECTS

10. Also we would apply the low electrical vibrations that may be had from the Radio-Active Appliance, that will make for the rest and for the overcoming of those conditions where the disturbances arise that prevent the body from resting or recuperating as it should in its proper periods of rest. We would attach this each day, preferably just before retiring, for at least thirty minutes to an hour; or, if it's necessary at other periods, it may be taken for a short period, but it will be found to be making for a balancing of the nerve energies and of the blood supply necessary for the replenishing and rebuilding throughout the system.

11. We would also use the *Violet Ray*; not the ultra-violet but the hand *Violet Ray*, preferably the hand charge and not the bulb variety, you see. This we would take about the body much in the same way as the Radio-Active Appliance would be attached; that is, one day it would be taken through the right hand and the next day through the left hand; the next day through the right foot and the next day through the left foot, and so circulate about the body. For these vibrations will make for charges in the system that will so stimulate the activities of that released by the raising of the subluxations in the areas indicated as to make for the proper balance throughout the system. It is well that these be taken until there is felt and breathed in much of the ozone created by such an activity; hence would be taken from twelve to fifteen minutes each day. Whether this treatment is given in the afternoon or evening does not matter. If it makes for a continuation of the treatment with the Radio-Active Appliance, it does not matter; for they are as a combination one with the other. 811-1/Spine:Subluxations/

****

3. The BLOOD SUPPLY shows rather poor eliminations, or the poor activity of the flow from the liver as accorded with the balancing of the gastric flow in the system - or a tendency for acidity through the non-activity of the gall ducts. This makes the mucus membranes of the circulation to the head, through the secondary cardiac plexus area, susceptible to congestion or cold; which forms or produces an over supply of lymph to the bronchi and larynx area, producing an irritation that makes for a deep, hoarse or heavy cough [Here Mr. Cayce imitated the cough]. So, there are produced in the system reflex conditions, or the tendencies for the acidity to attack more of the flow from the ducts or lacteals and lachrymal ducts; so that at times we have overflows from the eyes that make for irritations, and from the nostrils - also attacking the salivary glands, so that there is the congestion taken again through the gastric flow which makes for congestion through the inability of the system to digest properly.

7. Also the application of the Violet Ray (hand machine with bulb applicator) over throat and chest, for periods of three to four minutes every day - or twice a day is not too much for the present condition - would be very helpful. Do these, as we find in the present; and unless other conditions arise we will rid the conditions within the system. Not only by the effect of the medicinal properties internally but the effect upon the ganglia by the applications of the massage, that will affect directly the flow of the lymph or superficial circulation with lymph through the ganglia of the area, and then the stimulations to all the muscular forces through the *Violet Ray* - for the ozone that arises from same (which at times will not be so pleasant to the body) will be most beneficial, if it is inhaled. 566-3 /Cold Congestion/

****

DIZZY SPELLS

3. Now, the body shows improvement throughout, through the application of those conditions as have been given. While we find that the gold, with the diet as has been used for the body, has not reacted to the eliminations in the proper way and manner, this produced, as seen, by the diet. The vibratory forces, as is set by the application of the *Violet Ray*, have proven beneficial throughout. The reaction as produced - those dizzy spells - is from the non-elimination centers being stimulated by this vibratory force, in liver, spleen, and in the intestinal system. Hence, we would use now, added to these, those properties as will produce more eliminations - not leaving off the gold, or the vibratory forces in *Violet Ray*, in the manner as has been given, but keep away from those diets that cause fermentation in the intestinal tract, through the lower portion, through the colon, and through that portion of the body. Rather those to bring the laxative forces, and the elimination, with a stimulation to the liver, see? These, we find, would be in more GREEN vegetable forces, see? No meats - not too much broths, or things of that nature. Beef JUICES may be used, but NOT the MEATS, see?
464-2 /Toxemia, Glands, Incoordination/

****

3. (Q) Why does the gold and *Violet Ray* cause weakness and dizziness?
(A) These do not of themselves cause weakness and dizziness. Does the body desire [If the body desires] that the condition be improved, these must be applied in the way and manner given; that is, have gold in the system and the assimilation taking place when the *Violet Ray* vibrations are applied to the body, for this becomes necessary in that same way and manner as a purgative causes dizziness and sickness of stomach when there is congestion in liver. In the nerve centers as are acted upon by the active principle of gold in the system, functioning with the glands that give rejuvenation to all of the system, these being in that state of abnormal, or below normal, in their activity, the vibration set up by the action of electrical forces produces dizziness. This stood for a little, will bring conditions to the body, will the body [if the body will] apply same, see?
464-4 /Glands, Incoordination/

****

3. Thus pressures have been produced upon the nervous system, so as to prevent the body from relaxing perfectly when attempting to sleep; making restlessness or insomnia, producing headaches; that become very detrimental or terrifying to the portions of the head especially above the ears and across the top, the back of the neck and the like.
4. And sometimes the digestive system is upset, until it becomes dizzy and nauseated.
5. As we find for this body, the Hydrotherapy Bath would be well; which would be to lie in great quantities or a tub of water for a long period - this being kept a little above the temperature of the body; then followed by a thorough massage by a masseuse. This would be better than adjustments OR deep treatments, though it will be found that with the massage along the spine, with the body prone upon the face, these would - with the knuckle on either side of the spinal column - tend to make many a segment come nearer to normalcy, by being so treated AFTER having been thoroughly relaxed for twenty to thirty minutes IN the warm or hot water, see?

6. These then would be followed of evening by a little general electrical treatment, not too much; which might be had from the *Violet Ray*; or, better still, the Radio-Active Appliance - or a very low form of battery appliance - this directly to the body. As we find, the Radio-Active Appliance would be better than the others. But the *Violet Ray* may be taken in moderation, if chosen - the direct current from the *Violet Ray* along the spine, just before retiring.   635-9/Insomnia: Headaches/

ELIMINATIONS & STIMULATION

7. Through that of the osteopathic forces in system, in conjunction with electrical forces in *Violet Ray* over the centers that receive the incentive for stimulating the excretory functioning of the body, and by taking in the system properties in that of soda and gold, in this quantity:

8. To 15 ounces of distilled water add 10 grains Chloride of Gold and 15 grains of Bicarbonate of Soda. Shake well together. The dose would be 5 drops in half a glass of water twice each day, morning and evening. This we will find will so enliven nerve tissue, and especially that in the creative plasmatic cells, and receive the greater enlivenment or incentive through the *Violet Ray*, and give each in its action in system the incentive to eliminate used forces and prevent the formation of that bacilli that produces inflammation in the system. Also stimulating the nerve and muscular tissue in right portion of body, so that the condition in other side of body will come to function nearer the normal condition. Also relieving pain in the body.

9. Then the osteopathic forces should be applied to the system every other day very full, every other day nearer the massage of muscular forces, that we may keep the centralization and proper eliminations set in this system, with the *Violet Ray* applied, not above the cervical, or above the first dorsal, but below and over all portions of the body twice each day, thirty minutes after the gold has been taken in the system. Let the application be with not too strong a current, but be applied for at least ten to fifteen minutes each day.   9-5 /Blindness/

****

2. Then, only those conditions as would be in an easy, simple diet - not an over amount of sweets or of stimulants, but that which will produce rather a laxative reaction to the whole of the ELIMINATING system, and the application of vibrations either in manipulation - or preferably both the massage (or manipulation) and the actinic or *Violet Ray* for the body. THESE will bring the nearer normal reactions for THIS system.   140-29 /Cold Susceptibility/

****

8. Apply the vibrations of the *Violet Ray* occasionally, that the eliminations may not become centralized in any of the joints, or in portions of the system where distresses come through this toxin.   287-5 /Toxemia/

****

10. For those tendencies of the gathering of influences in system, and of the pneumatic or rheumatic condition, it would be well that the large quantities of the electro-magnetic or *Violet Ray* be applied to the superficial portions of the body, or that there be the charging of the body throughout with same, so as to reduce the salts and allow the eliminations to be carried from the system. 287-11 / Rheumatism: Tendancies/

****

11. The osteopathic treatments and adjustments may be made with a few minutes treatment after same with the *Violet Ray*, at not too high a discharge. [*Violet Ray* hand machine, bulb applicator.] DO that as given, if we would bring the bettered conditions for the body. Do as we have given. It is NECESSARY that the basis, or that which produces the condition, be corrected - for without this the local applications mean treating only effects and NOT the cause. The heat must be applied, and the stimuli of nerve reaction in *Violet Ray* is as necessary as any portion. 302-7 /Spine: Subluxations/

****

6. So, three or four days after the X-Ray treatment begin with the *Violet Ray* hand machine (rather than the ultra-violet). To be sure, this is objectionable to the body, but if the bulb is placed on the body and THEN the current turned on - GENTLY - this will NOT be objectionable. It is necessary to start eliminations, and to keep them maintained to overcome this tendency for the accumulations in the stomach of the forces that should be carried from the system - and that cause the inability for the food values to be taken. 325-06 /Cancer/

****

2. Now, as we find, there are very troublesome conditions in the physical forces of this body. These have been the outgrowth of minor disorders at first; and the neglect of the care respecting the eliminations brought about the thinning of the walls in the blood supply as related to the lymph circulation, producing those conditions first of the nature of swellings in portions of the body. Later these have taken on more of the ARTHRITIC tendencies. And adhesions have been made in portions of the system that have affected the locomotion, especially in the lower portions of the body; the UPPER portion having adjusted itself somewhat to the general conditions, though still affecting the body in part.

6. On those days when the above oil rub is not given, it would be well to use first warm packs of plain salt; preferably the heavy coarse salt heated in bags and placed along the spine, massaging THROUGH the salt packs gently along the spine and also on the limbs - not to produce irritation; but the heat IN the sacks AND the massage will be the aid. Afterwards apply the *Violet Ray* (hand machine, bulb applicator) over the same areas, and across the abdomen and down from the area of the diaphragm (right and left across the body), then down over the liver and over the caecum and up and across the colon area and down, following the outline across the abdomen, see? 676-1 /Arthritis/

****

5. Also, the use of the *Violet Ray* will make for the nerves' reaction in the cerebrospinal system to be more active, more effective. 4143-1/Neurasthenia/

****

12. (Q) How often should the *Violet Ray* be applied, and how long at a time?
(A) This should be applied rather consistently with the conditions. As understood by the body, in its analyses of physical reaction, the reaction of a physical body is as necessary for the full correction as for the applications that will bring relief at any period. So, the use of the *Violet Ray* should be consistent; not to give excess stimulation but to make for those reactions that bring the stimuli of the circulation both in nerve and blood supply to the portions affected. Then, take as outlined for the balancing of the elementals in the system. If necessary, when the body is tired or when there has been strain, use for ten to fifteen minutes each day; or if necessary use more than once a day, but when unnecessary do not become dependent upon its reactions for the feelings; rather work the physical body to that condition where the responses are from within self - see?   4143-1/Neurasthenia/

****

9. Applying each evening, after the bath, those of the *Violet Ray* over the extremities - especially the bottoms of the feet, palms of the hands, armpits, across the groin, across the lower portion of the abdomen. This will so stimulate the nerve centers and plexus from which the radiation is to the whole system, as to create a different vibration.   5525-1/Arthritis/

****

5. (Q) Constipation...?
(A) With the amount of changes as is indicated in the system with the change of secretion from the spleen will aid the paustolic [peristaltic] movements of the system. Regards gas action of the oxygen of the decomposed carbon, will release same by the application of the *Violet Ray*, this will reduce the amount of gas and increase secretion throughout the intestinal system.
5685-1/Assimilations: Eliminations/

****

4. (Q) Shall he keep up the use of the *Violet Ray*?
(A) WELL that these vibrations be kept for the system, also that the diets as have been given be kept near in the direction - though changes may be made from time to time in this direction to meet the changes in the physical forces as are being corrected in body. The *Violet Ray* application should be preferably AFTER the manipulations for the proper coordinating of the sympathetic and cerebro-spinal forces.
5. (Q) How often should the Violet Ray be used?
(A) Every other day, or the manipulations every other day and the *Violet Ray* EVERY day if not TOO long application of same. WELL, though, that this be applied while the body is relaxed from the manipulations.   195-58/Neurasthenia/
23. Give the Violet Ray each evening, FOLLOWING the massage. The massage need not necessarily be made as corrective measures osteopathically, but may be more in the nature of the neuropathic. Begin at the base of brain and go TOWARDS the central portion of body. Begin at the lower limbs and go (along the muscular forces on the inside, or following out the sciatic nerve centers along the inside of the limbs) to the trunk portion of body. Then along the cerebro-spinal system to the middle portion. Then we would give the *Violet Ray* for three to ten minutes each evening. This will so stimulate the circulation to the exterior portions, and vitalize the whole activities through an increased activity of the assimilated forces of the system, as to bring the proper balance in the body.   263-1/Anemia/

****

10. (Q) Would the *Violet Ray* be helpful?
(A) The *Violet Ray* will be helpful, provided there are those activities that make for sufficient assimilations that are helpful toward revitalizing the system. You see, the *Violet Ray* is only an electrical vibration that coordinates the vibratory forces of the bodily functioning itself - which means the circulation as related to the nerve forces of the body. Then, to revitalize the old blood cells without new being builded makes for a deterioration quick with same and becomes detrimental rather than helpful. But to have these to coordinate together, or to have the rebuilding and THEN the revitalizing, it is as the addition of strength to the body under such conditions. 1187-9/Apoplexy: After Effects/

****

10. We would use the Hand *Violet Ray*; this for the nerve forces will aid especially, if it is GRADUALLY used across the abdominal area; this given just before the body retires, or when it is prepared for rest of evenings, will aid in better rest and will aid in relaxing the body and stimulating better eliminations. Take about fifteen minutes in making the application; not going through it hurriedly, but each portion to which it is applied given due consideration. Use the bulb applicator, so that it may be used as a character of massage; along the spine - but HERE, ALWAYS downward, NEVER the strokes upward! and also across the abdomen, slowly. Though there will be some interference and some resistance to this, at first, we find that it may gradually be used. Across the abdomen it would be rather as a kneading or a massaging. Fifteen minutes in all. And we will find this to be a most helpful portion of the treatments in the present. 1553-2 /Senility/

****

5. We would find much improvement and it much better for the body to take the *Violet Ray* as indicated, when the body is ready to retire. For the reactions upon the body of this being given with the periods of manipulation and adjustment DO NOT work as well as if they were separate - or given more often; not necessarily deep, but the activities of these would be more in keeping with that for helpful forces and would make the body rest much better. 1563-2/Toxemia/

****

21. Also we would use the low vibrations from the *Violet Ray* (hand machine, bulb applicator), when there is the tendency towards tiredness in the limbs, through the shoulders, and the heaviness through the abdominal area. Do not give it too strong, but for a minute and a half apply the bulb applicator along the spine - when ready to retire. It will make those centers corrected (by the mechanical means, or osteopathically) coordinate with the juices, especially of beets, in the body. We would use the *Violet Ray* two, three to four times a week; this dependent upon the feeling of the body, you see. Use just before retiring. The body may use the applicator itself or have it applied by one close to the body at the time, see? 2946-1/Arthritis/

****

4. There should be those manipulations and corrections in the cerebro-spinal system, that will alleviate the pressures in the lumbar and dorsal region, as well as alignments in the upper dorsal and cervical. These should be taken, as we would find, at least three to four times each week. These may be given either osteopathically or chiropractically, so that the ADJUSTMENTS or the alleviations are made.
5. Then, after each treatment, there should be the vibrations from the *Violet Ray* for at least three to

four, to five minutes, over the WHOLE of the cerebrospinal system, to enliven the circulation OVER the centers that especially are adjusted.   5493-1/Spine: Subluxations/

****

3. As we would find in the present, each day there should be a general stimulation with the *Violet Ray* along the upper dorsal and upper cervical, or throughout the cervical area; around the neck and the head, around the ear; and then a general massage - not a treatment but a massage, as with the electrically driven vibrator. These would continue to make for greater improvements in the general physical forces of the body.   413-5/Tinnitus/

****

17. (Q) What type of electrical appliance should be used, and how often?
(A) The *Violet Ray*. This the body may apply to self, or have applied to self at home; for it should be given, and will be better for the stimulations to the system through this be given each evening for three to fifteen minutes, over the cerebro-spinal system and, specifically, in the locomotory centers, the brachial centers, and those tautnesses that occur occasionally in the head and neck.
446-1/Eliminations: Incoordination/

****

16. After some six or eight adjustments have been taken, begin also with the *Violet Ray* (hand machine) as a direct application. First, use the bulb applicator from the lower portion of the spine to the areas about the head and neck, - along each side of the spine, and such an application should last some three minutes.   2638-1/Cataracts/

****

3. Then, to bring about the more normal condition for this body, we would, through those deep manipulations, osteopathically given, correct those conditions in the cerebrospinal system, and at the same time apply the vibration from the *Violet Ray* over the whole cerebrospinal nerve system. That is, as the body is adjusted and treated, osteopathically, the next day, or two days, each day lie prone on face and apply the vibrations from the *Violet Ray* direct to the cerebro- spinal system, beginning at the upper cervicals and following out each center and its branches along the spine. As is seen, head and neck - then the arms and shoulders - then the whole torso, and along the whole length of each sciatic nerve, and especially along the channel, or route, as it were, of each branch of the sympathetic nerve system, treating the body in such a manner for twenty-five to thirty-five minutes at least four times each week.   2672-1/Eyes-Lesions/

Please note that the currently manufactured Violet Ray hand held unit instructions recommend using no more than 10 minutes at a time before the unit must be allowed to cool.

****

13. R E L I E F, to give the relief to this body, and to bring the normal condition, and to prevent the further conditions in the capillary circulation, the poor elimination, or centers from becoming broken in the cell building force, and to produce the elimination and assimilation proper, we would first adjust those conditions in the dorsal and lumbar region, applying then with this, after the first four adjustments or manipulation for adjustments, as given, those as found in the *Violet Ray* over the whole system.

14. Do that, and we will find within six to ten weeks the body perfectly normal from these conditions.

15. (Q) How often should the *Violet Ray* treatment be given?

(A) Every day for five minutes. After the fifth treatment in the deep manipulation and adjustments for these vibrations to become effective in nerve system and in the circulation of the capillary circulation. 4359-01 /Eliminations/

****

2. Now, when these properties as have been given [in 236-1] in the entirety have been completed, we would rest from same five (5) days. Then have this prepared and begin and take another full quantity - beginning, however, AT ONCE, with the use of the Violet Ray. With the body lying prone (on face), just before retiring, follow out the whole cerebro-spinal nervous system, beginning at the base of the brain, going slowly to the full length of the spine, retracing slowly in the same manner and way, using the bulb - the larger bulb. After this has been gone over four, five, to six times, slowly, each center, then follow out the line of the brachial plexus, along arms, see? Then down to the solar plexus, and this rather heavy. Then from that of the sciatic nerves, or the lower plexus - locomotary plexus, down each limb, see? under side, or with the body lying prone - just this portion.

3. We find this, kept up each evening for at least thirty (30) days, will show the difference in the blood and in the nerve reaction, ridding the system of nerve headaches, assisting in digestion and assimilation, and stimulating all of the circulatory system to a near normal property. 236-2 / Eliminations/Assimilation /

COMMON COLD SUSCEPTIBILITY

1. EC: Now, we find there are some conditions that are different from those when we had this here before. Some are better. Others we find congestion has brought about different conditions in different portions of the body. We only need to keep more of the vibration that is made through the manipulation [osteopathic, by Dr. Wm. A. Gravett, D.O.] and the medicinal properties for those portions of the system, and it is necessary that the vibrations of the *Violet Ray* be given, that the body may receive the equalization of the circulation and the assimilation in nerve centers and action, that the body may resist more than it has been, for under such conditions does the congestion, as at present, to the tissue of the larynx, bronchials and nasal cavities and tissue show how the congestion may react upon system. 538-7/Cold: Congestion/

****

7. Thus the hindering or slowing of the circulation has made for definite conditions that are now aggravating to the bronchi and larynx area; thus producing a little hacking cough which only at times causes any great amount of phlegm to be raised from the throat or lungs - when there has been an excess of cold or congestion.

11. All of these as we find are rather of a sympathetic nature and of a general run-down condition for the body.

20. Each evening, just before retiring, apply the Violet Ray (hand machine, bulb applicator) for three minutes along either side of the spine.

27. All of these we would keep in their regular order as indicated, - the periods of adjustments, the periods of rest during which we would use the Violet Ray and the massage, etc. When the body begins to feel better, do not quit. There will be periods of a great deal of help, and at other periods there will be seemingly some irritation - but keep these up, for we will correct the general health, retard the loss of vision, and aid in bringing bettered conditions for the body.   2417-1/Congestion/

****

14. The vibration of *Violet Ray* should be accorded the whole system, especially over feet and the lower limbs, along the sciatic nerves and across the sacral and in the plexus of the cervical and upper dorsal. Not so much in solar plexus region. Do this each evening. In five to six weeks we will find the body more active mentally and physically, and better fitted for physical activities.   137-1/Circulation/

NEURASTHENIA

"Neurasthenia is a neurosis affecting various organs and functions and characterized by ready and persistent exhaustibility and increased nervous irritability. It is caused by organic disease, such as tuberculosis, arteriosclerosis, diabetes, etc." Medical Diseases for Nurses, Stevens & Ambler.

11. We would also use the *Violet Ray* applicator, or the *Violet Ray* - using the bulb applicator, and beginning in the central portion of the spine treat DOWNWARD; that is, away from the heart, see, away from the upper circulation, to the end of the spine; then down to the toes, principally along the back portion of the limbs, along the sciatic, but particularly over the lumbar and sacral area. Beginning at the 8th or 9th dorsal, go downward each way for FIFTEEN minutes. Do not use the *Violet Ray* ABOVE the diaphragm area, but DOWNWARD - and AWAY FROM the body. This may be given each evening at the time for retirement, see?   483-1/Neurasthenia/

****

4. (Q) Shall he keep up the use of the Violet Ray?

(A) WELL that these vibrations be kept for the system, also that the diets as have been given be kept near in the direction - though changes may be made from time to time in this direction to meet the changes in the physical forces as are being corrected in body. The Violet Ray application should be preferably AFTER the manipulations for the proper coordinating of the sympathetic and cerebro-spinal forces.

5. (Q) How often should the Violet Ray be used?

(A) Every other day, or the manipulations every other day and the Violet Ray EVERY day if not TOO long application of same. WELL, though, that this be applied while the body is relaxed from the manipulations.   195-58 / Neurasthenia /

****

2. While conditions are somewhat changed from that as we have had here before, conditions are not good at all. For the body overtaxes itself physically, and disregards - often - the effect of food values being taken when there are mental and physical anxieties. Hence we have a very DEPLETED blood supply, a very strained nerve system.

6. Keep the low electrical vibrations. These are preferable to superficial circulation. The plain Violet Ray, you see. This will REST the body. This should be given from the back of the head to the sole of the feet, and this should be given NOT STRONG - but gentle, to relax the body.

18. (Q) What is the cause and cure for the soreness on the right side of my head?

(A) The poor circulation, and the general activities of the system would be necessary to relieve same; or the specific activity of the general application of the Violet Ray over the whole system. This will relax the system sufficient to change the circulation, so as to prevent the poor circulation and the poor nerve energies from localizing.

19. (Q) What time of the day would the Violet Ray be best used?

(A) Just before retiring!   307-10 / Strained Nervous System /

MENOPAUSE (MENORRHAGIA)

The cessation of menstruation.

13. After the Tonicine has been taken for a week, and at least two adjustments, we would begin then (not before) with the use of the *Violet Ray* (hand machine); but we would use this a little bit differently from the manner ordinarily used. Do not use the bulb applicator, but rather the ROD applicator; and use it first with the right hand, the next day with the left foot - but lay the anode or applicator upon glass, then place the foot upon same. The next day use the applicator in the left hand, then the next day the right foot placed upon same - after it is laid on the glass; and so on about the body. Do this each day for at least ten days. Then leave this off until the second series of the osteopathic treatments, then take again. Do not take this longer than two minutes in the first series, or longer than three minutes in the second series, see?   1540-3/Menopause/

****

1. EC: There is much difference in the physical conditions in this body since last we had it. Some of these are better conditions, some have been created from the same conditions. Others have arisen by the change in the cycle of the physical developments [Menopause?], and by conditions as have been produced through action and counter-action in the system.

17. Then every third day apply the low vibration of the *Violet Ray* over extremities, and the whole length of spine, with the body lying prone on its face. [*Violet Ray* hand machine, bulb applicator.]
325-3/Eliminations:Poor/

****

8. Those periods of the nominal reaction to the nervous system (the menopause) are not set in their reaction to the body.

9. Hence we find (though such periods are long passed, as nominal) the nervous disturbance, the inability for proper digestion, the tendencies for the insomnia, the tendencies for the body to become easily excited; the activities through the whole system of heaviness in the extremities, and the imaginative forces becoming as a part of the physical reaction, become part and parcel of the whole disturbance for the body.

16. We would use each day for one hour, just before retiring of an evening, the Radio-Active Appliance. This as we find will equalize the circulation and tend to make the body able to rest without sediments or sedatives of any kind. This should be kept very clean - that is, the plates or anodes - and attached to opposite sides of the body; right wrist, left ankle; left wrist, right ankle. In the preparation have the Appliance in the ice, not so much water, and do not allow the water or the ice in the crock container (not a metal) to come over the top of the Appliance at any time. Put the Appliance in the ice fifteen minutes before it is attached to the body, or the leads attached to same to attach to the body. Let the Appliance remain in the ice, of course, during the whole period of application. This we would find to be most helpful.

17. Also we would use the Violet Ray, but not strong - and not more than half a minute in the beginning. There may be the tendencies at times for this to irritate the body, but if it is given it will be found to be helpful. Preferably use the bulb applicator along the spine, if possible - but this must be applied directly to the body itself, to be sure; gently massaging downward and especially across the lumbar area, across the solar plexus centers or area and across the shoulders and the head and neck; but not more than a minute or three-quarters of a minute in the beginning. If the bulb applicator is found to be impractical, then use the rod applicator that is held only in the hand - or may be placed on a glass and the foot put on same, see? and if this is used, alternate - once in the hand, the next time upon the foot and the opposite side of the body; or alternate - right foot, then the left hand; left hand, then just the opposite, you see - on the foot - continuing about the body in this way. However, it is preferable to use the bulb applicator if possible.   1343-2 / Menopause

****

14. (Q) Why is pulse so rapid at times?
(A) As just indicated, this is the effect of the disturbance through the upper hepatic circulation; which causes a quick return or flow as it were of the circulatory forces from the heart to the liver; quickening the pulse as well as the nerve tension in the periods that are preceding the menopause.
15. (Q) Is this why the menstrual period is irregular?
(A) This is a portion of the disturbance.
16. (Q) What is trouble in left ovary?
(A) The inclination for the poisons, or a sympathetic effect from the poisons from the system. Hence,

as indicated, the necessity of cleansing first the alimentary canal and stimulating more normalcy in the hepatic circulation, as well as using the douches to purify the conditions through the pelvic organs and their activities. This should aid a great deal. Of course, the use of the electrically driven vibrator over the body of evenings would be especially helpful in equalizing and causing a better circulatory force; especially using the sponge applicator across the abdomen and pelvis, and even across the lower portion of the lumbar area.

17. (Q) Should Codiron be continued and for how long?

(A) This we would continue, especially through the winter and early spring.

18. (Q) Should *Violet Ray* be continued - and how?

(A) This may be used occasionally, and especially to quiet the nerves; through the shoulders and neck and head, across the diaphragm area and through the spine and limbs.
313-17/Cholecystitis Tendencies/

****

3. In the blood supply, we find these conditions at the present time: the blood itself being and is carrying many properties that should be eliminated in the system other than as being eliminated at the present time, produced first by properties of the potash nature taken in system to produce a nerve relaxing and coming in contact with conditions in system, and properties as taken in system as foods working in opposition to each other affect the kidneys and the liver in their eliminating functioning. Also with the age [beginning of menopause?] and the condition existing in the pelvic organs, in that known as the menstrual periods being and acting under the strain of the condition, produces a taxing in eliminating centers, especially in blood supply gives the overcharges to be eliminated. These conditions working in conjunction then produce in various portions of the body the rash or eliminating through capillary circulation poisons that should be carried through dross either in intestinal tract or through the emunctories and eliminated through the urine. This is better that the condition exists externally than that the organs should become defective and produce the condition on the organs, kidneys, liver, [She died 4/1/45 of carcinoma of liver.], stomach or lungs, than the condition be there and produce the same effects internally as shown externally; yet conditions may be turned so that proper elimination may be created in the system and in the correct manner remove these drosses and dregs from system, without the system becoming so distressing and so terrifying to the capillaries and external nerve system. This we find also is controlled, as given, great deal by nerve plexus and centers, for the body, as has been given, is of the neurotic [See 538-55, etc.] temperament or tendency.

4. In the nerve system, the condition at present we find many centers involved in conditions, yet all very much better under the control of the mental forces of body, and of the physical functioning of organs, than when we had the condition before.

5. In the functioning of organs:

6. Brain forces very good. Needs to keep the subjugation of mental forces under that control of the soul and spirit forces necessary to keep an equilibrium in the sympathetic nerve system. The plexuses in the solar plexus, the secondary cardiac plexus, the second lumbar plexus show how strain is on system and how the functioning through these, the sudden appearance or the attempt of the nerve system to assist circulation to eliminate, and those portions that come closest to the emunctory circulation suffer first, as this condition under arms, in and about the pelvic organs and the pubes, especially forearms and the portions where lymphatic is closest to the capillary circulation. Heat or cold, either excitement or depression, brings to the sympathetic system the sudden reaction and the best forces are exercised through the control of the mental attributes of the physical. In the nose,

nostril, the condition exists as we have had before. The effects in the nerve reaction not so prominent as has been in times back, due to circulation and system in nerve forces attempting to make correct adjustments. Lungs much better than we have had before. Stomach and upper portion of digestion not good, yet better than before. The secretions as given in system from a torpid liver, a high hepatic circulation, though a cold one and the hypogastric in its depression through circulation in blood and in nerve ganglion both show the contraction and the lack of proper secretions being produced in system. Then, in lower digestion, we find still more effects as of this same condition as created through the hypogastric plexus and the effect produced on the hepatic circulation. Kidneys in much better condition than when we had them before.

7. Then to bring the relief to this body, we must bring those conditions to bear and the body must be persistent and consistent with the conditions to be met with the treatment accorded same. For the condition we would keep properties as being taken; that of the sulphur and cream of tartar, or phosphates in that form, adding charcoal and the secretions forming as we would find in Epsom Salts in a consistent form. In these quantities take one charcoal tablet each day, preferably in evening. Take two small doses of Epsom Salts each day, one morning, one evening. The condition as is found in vagina and in the pubes, [vaginitis & pruritis vulvae] where the irritation from discharge [leukorrhea], and from nerve condition, we would use the spiral douches, the solution as would be given in Permanganate of Potash, with equal small quantities of Myrrh. Also using sitz-baths every second day, as this: Into a gallon and a half of very warm water, add 5 drops Tincture of Myrrh, 10 grains Balsam of Tolu. Sit over this in a basin and expose parts where itching is so terrifying to the body. For the douches, use Permanganate just sufficient that the water may show the color - just a few drops. The Myrrh, one to two minims, using this once each day. This does not interfere with other as is used. For the condition on the cuticle, only keep such properties as will prevent the body from becoming too irritated, such as dusted with Stearate of Zinc with the Balsam, and keep the bowels acting properly. Keep from the diet of properties that excite too much of the functioning of the organs in the form of astringents. That is, not too much acids in any form, until an equalization is created.

8. Do that. We will bring the normal conditions to this body, [538].

9. (Q) Should the *Violet Ray* treatment be continued?
(A) This strengthens any vibration and is good for the nerve system, when alcohols in no form are taken. Detrimental when used or in or on any portion of the body. The electrode for the vagina is very good, and when taken should be left in for several minutes. There should be no exciting of the genital organs [sexually, etc.?], until the system has at least reached its equilibrium, in any manner or form.
538-8/Vaginitis/

*The Violet Ray electrodes for internal use are not available today. Electrodes are **NOT** for internal use!
****

12. (Q) Why is there inflammation about the breast?
(A) As just indicated, the incoordination of the glandular forces of the system; and this, as the changes are coming about in the system, [Menopause?] is affecting the mammary glands, see?
13. (Q) May an affirmation be given to be used in administering the massage?
(A) The affirmation would be more effective if used with the Radio-Active Appliance when IT is used. For this is nearer in accord with the activities of the coordination between the physical, mental and spiritual forces of the body itself. For when these are mechanically done, or through individuals, these make for then a different character of current that naturally coordinates or works through the body. Hence at such periods when the Radio-Active Appliance is used, let the affirmation be as this - but put in the words of the individuals themselves:

LET THERE BE PERFORMED IN MY BODY THAT SERVICE, THAT ACTIVITY O FATHER, THOU SEEST NECESSARY TO MAKE MY BODY WHOLE; THAT I MAY BE THE GREATER SERVICE FOR THEE IN THIS EXPERIENCE.

The words, of course, may be altered, but let them be with that purpose, that intent.

14. (Q) What causes me to be so fatigued after talking, and what can be done for same?

(A) This is a reaction to the sensory forces of the body, and should be much bettered as there are the adjustments osteopathically for the general circulation and for the relieving of the nerve pressure.

15. (Q) What causes weakness in back?

(A) The same as has just been indicated.

16. (Q) Would an electric vibrator be helpful?

(A) This as we find would be rather severe. If there would be taken electricity itself, we find it would be better; in a very low form, as in the *Violet Ray* - but not with the bulb, rather with the hand or rod applicator, see? Not too high nor for too long. Half a minute once a day should be sufficient in the beginning. These treatments would also be more effective if alternated about the body; that is: The first day hold the rod in the right hand, the next day lay the applicator on a piece of glass and set the left foot on it and then turn on the electricity. The next day hold it in the left hand, the next day use it with the right foot. Keep alternating the applications about the body in this manner.

560-6/Cancer: Breasts/

****

2. Now, as we find, there are conditions that disturb the better physical functioning of the body. These have to do with the eliminations and the changes that are naturally coming about in the physical forces of the body at this time.

3. The affectations, then, are to the nervous systems of the body and the reaction upon the physical organisms in their functioning.

4. These, then, are conditions as we find them with this body, [865] we are speaking of:

5. In the BLOOD SUPPLY, here we find the indications of the disturbances in the physical forces, as well as in the functioning organs and the lack of a normal or nominally equalized circulation, owing to the periods or the menopause being in the activities of the system. Hence we have periods of headaches, tiredness, the feet and lower limbs giving distress through overactivity or of being too quiet in some portions of the cycle of the activity. These are but the effects of the nervous disturbance and the attempts of the body to adjust itself to the changes in the activities of the system.

6. The blood supply itself is somewhat low in the necessary forces to make for a normalcy in supplying sufficient of the nutriment for the upbuilding. Hence we have, from this same disturbance, periods of the inability for proper rest, and those reactions that arise from same.

18. The use of the *Violet Ray* as a portion of the treatment two or three times each week, especially over the lumbar, the solar plexus and brachial plexus center, will be helpful or beneficial. This should be added preferably just before retiring. 865-1/Menopause/

****

2. As we find, there are disturbing conditions in the physical forces of the body. These as we find, in their basic condition, arise from specific disturbances; but the reactions in the system with the changes that are and have been gradually coming about, or the beginnings of the periods of menopause, are changed or altered.

3. Hence we have those continued periods of headaches, indigestion, disturbance with eliminations,

the overnervous spells; and periods when there are hot and cold sensations.

4. These are effects, not causes; and, other than just a help, there needs to be those proper corrections made as would alleviate the causes of the disturbance and - during these periods of transition in physical functioning - make for the conditions becoming nominal or normal for the body.

7. Hence we have periods when it becomes necessary that there be a purifying of same by such increased eliminations as to produce greater strain upon that basic cause of the disturbance.

18. After at least four or five of the complete adjustments osteopathically are made, we would use the *Violet Ray* of an evening before retiring, to soothe the nerve forces of the body. Begin at the base of the brain, a circular motion along either side of the cerebrospinal system, extending all the way to the lower portion of the spine; then down the sciatic nerve to the bottoms of the feet. Do this for periods of a week to two weeks, rest from same a few days (not weeks, but days), and then begin again.   1342-1/Menopause/

LARYNGITIS

"Laryngitis is an inflammation of the laryngeal mucosa and is due to bacterial or oral infection which results in a partial or complete loss of voice. Hoarseness is the main symptom." Edgar Cayce Encyclopedia of Healing

2. In the present the cold, congestion that has existed in the lungs, larynx, bronchials, in the head, has taxed the system such as to cause the hoarseness; produced by the larynx and vocal cords being taut, through the inflammation and congestion exhibited there, the poisons from same in the system producing the disturbances through the alimentary canal.

3. Then, in the present, there may be either the increase of the circulation by magnetic influences or through the application of heat, with the vibrations of electrical forces in the *Violet Ray* over the area, or through the COMBINED application of these with suggestion.

4. We would also have the body refrain from smoking entirely until, at least, the congestion has been removed.

5. Keep a fruit and vegetable diet only, with the alkalin reaction in same.   294-165/Bronchitis/

VIOLET RAY AND RADIO-ACTIVE APPLIANCE, RADIAC©

*The Radio Active Appliance is now trademarked as the RADIAC® and is available through Baar Products, Inc. (1-800-269-2502)

24. The emotions of the body, as here, are as electronic energies. This again is a name, until the individual entity experiences that there is the heart beat and pulsation, there IS the respiratory activity of the lungs to purify the body-flow of life, blood, fluid, WITH a glow from the emotions controlled through the centers or lines of the nervous systems for both positive and negative natures.

25. There are those influences without the entity of those natures also. These have been indicated as necessary influences in the experience of this body, as an application, [263-12] through the use of the Violet Ray. This is a high voltage, stimulating all centers that are as the crossroads, the connections between the various portions of the physical-body functioning, the mental attitudes and attainments, as well as the sources of supply; which arose by the choice of the entity in entering this particular temple, this individual temple.

27. But, once in seven days apply the high vibrations with the Violet Ray. Take same not just to be gotten through with, but begin in the central portion of the nervous system - or the 9th dorsal - work upward to the brain, or base of brain, the head. Then go down on either side of the spine, then down to the end of the spine, even to the sciatic along the lower limbs and to the soles of the feet. Then back, either side, to the central portion. Take at least two minutes, three minutes, to accomplish this. Let it be in contact with the body.

28. Then at other periods, if necessary twice a day, use the very LOW electrical forces of the body itself, as may be exercised by the use of that called the Radio-Active Appliance. This would not be slap-dab put together, but in order, in decency and in order, and used as an equalizer, a stimulator to the general forces of the body as it COORDINATES.

29. Then apply the WILL in those things indicated. Ye KNOW the way. Then if ye are tired, if ye are tempestuous, within yourself, rest and apply the Radio-Active Appliance for twenty minutes of morning, twenty minutes in the afternoon - if necessary.   263-13 / Coordination /

****

11. We would also use the *Violet Ray*; not the ultra-violet but the hand *Violet Ray*, preferably the hand charge and not the bulb variety, you see. This we would take about the body much in the same way as the Radio-Active Appliance would be attached; that is, one day it would be taken through the right hand and the next day through the left hand; the next day through the right foot and the next day through the left foot, and so circulate about the body. For these vibrations will make for charges in the system that will so stimulate the activities of that released by the raising of the subluxations in the areas indicated as to make for the proper balance throughout the system. It is well that these be taken until there is felt and breathed in much of the ozone created by such an activity; hence would be taken from twelve to fifteen minutes each day. Whether this treatment is given in the afternoon or evening does not matter. If it makes for a continuation of the treatment with the Radio-Active Appliance, it does not matter; for they are as a combination one with the other.   811-1/Spine: Subluxations/

****

25. (Q) What causes and what should be done for the skin irritation, also the itching in ears?
(A) A low electrical vibration would be helpful for this -such as from the *Violet Ray*. There is a tendency for not exactly an eczema but an inclination in the direction. Leave off too much of the carbonated waters, and drinks with same. Use the *Violet Ray* about every other evening over the upper portion of the shoulders, the neck, the head; and we will find these conditions improving.

26. (Q) Is my Radio-Active Appliance still good?
(A) Only needs some little overhauling. But this electrical vibration as indicated is the *Violet Ray* that is needed, as well as the Radio-Active Appliance. This is the high vibration, while the Radio-Active is the vibratory force of the body set to work for making a more perfect circulation. The *Violet Ray* is the current carried directly into the system and is a destructive vibration, while the Radio-Active

vibration is constructive. These do not work in opposition to one another, but work on different portions of the system. The Ultra-Violet or the *Violet Ray* works upon the superficial circulation, while the low electrical vibration of the Radio-Active Appliance is an active principle with the deeper circulation - though it is taken in through the superficial. 416-12/Eczema/

****

13. We find that the use of the Radio-Active Appliance would be helpful in keeping the circulation equalized and in making for better rest for the body, enabling the body to sleep better. And, as is indicated with the use of the Radio- Active Appliance, when the body uses same for thirty minutes to an hour each day, it is well to remain quiet and in a meditative state of the mental reactions for the body. These will bring the more helpful conditions for the body.

14. A use of the hand *Violet Ray* occasionally on the back of the neck, from the base of the brain to the middle portion of the spine - or to the 9th dorsal, this applied as the body is ready to rest of an evening, will also make for a material aid in producing a quieting for the body. 774-4/Assimilations: Poor/

****

28. Begin immediately when these osteopathic treatments are begun, with the use of the *Violet Ray*. These vibrations may be taken at home, or just before retiring. A small portion of same should be applied about the head, the ear, the brachial center, the dorsal center, the lumbar center, and then across the diaphragm area. Then for three to five minutes just take the plain applicator (rod applicator) and hold in the hand.

29. We would also use the low electrical vibrations from the body through the Radio-Active Appliance, each evening before retiring - or when retiring. Attach on opposite extremities of the body, for creating the equalizations through the system. 1164-1/Assimilations: Eliminations: Incoordination/

****

3. As we find, while there are disturbances physically we find that these may be best met with the general attitude of the body if there are the body electrical forces applied; that is, with the Radio-Active Appliance. Use this for thirty minutes twice each day, and let those periods be set aside for prayer and meditation. Thus we will bring a better balance to these body forces. The frayed or weary nerve centers will be rejuvenated. The body forces and caused weakness in the limbs, will be much bettered.

4. Also each evening when ready to retire we would use, for about a minute and a half to two minutes, a gentle massage with a very low vibration of the *Violet Ray* (hand machine, bulb applicator). This will also assist in charging the centers of the body, as the equalizing is accomplished through the Radio-Active Appliance. This should be used along either side of the spine rather than directly on the spinal column itself, and along those areas that connect with the sciatic centers.
3264-1/Sciatica/

****

3. As we find, while there are disturbances physically we find that these may be best met with the general attitude of the body if there are the body electrical forces applied; that is, with the Radio-

Active Appliance. Use this for thirty minutes twice each day, and let those periods be set aside for prayer and meditation. Thus we will bring a better balance to these body forces. The frayed or weary nerve centers will be rejuvenated. The body forces and circulations, where irritations have caused weakness in the limbs, will be much bettered.

4. Also each evening when ready to retire we would use, for about a minute and a half to two minutes, a gentle massage with a very low vibration of the *Violet Ray* (hand machine, bulb applicator). This will also assist in charging the centers of the body, as the equalizing is accomplished through the Radio-Active Appliance. This should be used along either side of the spine rather than directly on the spinal column itself, and along those areas that connect with the sciatic centers.
483-1/Neurasthenia/

****

18. Hence we would use every day the Radio-Active Appliance, for a week or more. Then rest from same a few days, and then begin again. This would be most helpful and would REST the body. Or when the body is mentally or physically tired, even at other portions of the day, it will assist in making for resuscitating influences and be helpful in resting the body when it retires from physical activity. Keep the plates cleansed and the wires in perfect order. The attachments should be made, of course, to the opposite extremities.

19. Also in periods of two to three days at a time, with a rest from same for two or three days and then again, we would use in the evening when ready to retire a thorough treatment with the plain *Violet Ray* (hand machine, bulb applicator). This would be for recharging, as it were, the ganglia along the cerebro-spinal system. And especially would this be most helpful around the neck or throughout the cervical area, across those areas of the thyroid or the vagus nerve centers.
1049-1/Eliminations: Poor/

****

12. First, - we would use the body-force of the electrical treatments; as from the Radio-Active Appliance. Use this for a period of five to ten days at a time, then leave off for a week.

13. During that week it is left off, however, at least twice during the week have - when ready to retire, after the bath has been taken - the application of the *Violet Ray*; this to be along the spine, over the arms, shoulders, and over the limbs. Use the bulb applicator for this, but not turned on too high. This will give the "pick up" or the stimulation that is needed for what might be called the recharging of the centers along the cerebrospinal system, so that there is better coordination between the ganglia of the cerebrospinal and the sympathetic nerve system.   1196-17/Prostatitis: Toxemia/

****

10. Do occasionally, when tired from physical exercise, have either the ultra-violet or *Violet Ray* applied gently, or the electrically driven vibrator, or the Radio-Active Appliance. This will bring rest, it will bring the coordinating of the physical and the mental being.   1861-18/Lesions/

****

1. EC: Yes. Not so good are the conditions as we find with this body. We would use more of the vibrations from the Radio-Active Appliance, supplemented with the plain *Violet Ray*, adhering more to the diet and the applications along the cerebrospinal system - especially in those centers in the upper dorsal and cervical - that have been indicated in such conditions.   326-5/Neuralgia: Tendencies/

****

11. At least once each week when the osteopathic treatment is given (and there should be given at least two each week, with the manipulations and corrections), use with same in the treatment the plain *Violet Ray*.

12. Also we find that the use of the Radio-Active Appliance of evenings as the body rests will make for better coordination in the activities that are to be distributed by the manipulations. Apply this about thirty minutes each day, when the body rests in the afternoon or upon retiring in the evening. Make the connections first to the RIGHT wrist and then to the left ankle. The next day make the connection to the right ankle and to the left wrist; that is, making the connection at the ankle first, you see. In this way we will make the coordinations in a manner that will create an even balance mentally, physically, and give the spiritual reaction the better channel to function through.   577-1/
Glands: Incoordination/

****

16. After all of these have been given, then apply the *violet-ray*; beginning at the base of the brain, coming downward then, circular motion either side of the spinal system or along those connections specifically between the cerebro-spinal and the sympathetic nervous system. Let this be of a circular motion and keep on down to the 4th lumbar, then branch to a circular motion towards the plexus for the lower portion of the limbs. Extend this to the feet on either side and over the sciatic nerve center, under the knees, soles of the feet, the ankles and then from the feet back towards the body. This to carry nerve energies and stimulations.

17. After this has been given, let the body rest or be bathed off with a little rub alcohol, and then apply the Radio-Active Appliance to equalize circulation.
1195-2/Cancer: Tendencies/

****

13. In the whole of the system, these - as we find - may SOON be relieved, will those conditions be adhered to as will bring an alignment for the cerebrospinal nervous system, with any form of low electrical vibratory force that will aid the body in gaining a normal equilibrium in a nerve distorted center.

14. These, we find, would best be through the *Violet Ray*, used with the manipulations AND corrections for the cerebrospinal system, used during the same period, for three to five minutes.

15. Also, as the body rests, at least two or three times each week, use those low vibrations from the Radio-Active Appliance - PLAIN - attaching same in a circulatory manner; that is, right ankle, left wrist - left ankle, right wrist -in the anodes.   4091-1/Epilepsy/

EYES

The Double Eye Applicator is not available at this date. The general electrode or Bulb applicator can be used in its place.
• The eye lid must be closed when applying the bulb applicator.
• Never apply for more than 10 to 15 seconds
• Remove contact lenses before application.
• Do not use if you have lense implants.

9. (Q) What can I do to help the condition of my eyes as I have severe headaches the day after I read?
(A) This is another of those indications where the needs are for the deep manipulations in those specific areas as make for the associations of activities in the circulatory forces from those influences of the assimilating system. The reactions from the upper dorsal and throughout the cervical area from this character of treatment would relieve these pressures most perceptibly. We may get some stimulation also with the use of the *Violet Ray* in connection with the manipulative forces, but do not use same WITHOUT having the manipulative forces - for it would only make for a temporary reaction that would make for an aggravation of the condition later on. So, we would take two deep manipulative treatments each week for say three weeks; with special reference to the congested forces in the 3rd, 4th, 2nd, 1st dorsal and through the cervical area. Then once a week apply (by self) the *Violet Ray* (hand machine), using the double eye applicator. Do not use too long nor at too great a speed; but close the eyes, turn OFF the ray, and with it attached place the appliance or the anode or applicator over the eye and then GRADUALLY turn on - and only sufficient for the FEELING of the effect of these vibrations upon the eyes themselves. Then the next morning after these vibrations have been used (and the applicator would not remain on longer than a minute, you see), cleanse the eyes with a weak solution of an antiseptic nature that may make for the clearing of the eyes themselves. The eyewash as Murine is very good, or the Acids [Boracic Acid?] that are of a mild form are very good, or the Lavoris - though we would use it only half strength. These we find would be most helpful.
338-5/Lesions/

****

2. (Q) What further osteopathic treatments should body take from Dr. Berger to help his eyes improve?
(A) Added with those of the *Violet Ray*, with the double applicator directly to the eyes, with the drainages set up for those portions of the circulation through the central nervous system, especially following out those from the 1st and 2nd dorsal, 3rd, 4th and 5th cervical, to the upper side of the face - these will be helpful. As to how much, this will depend upon how much is necessary? How much will he take? How much does he want? Follow those. Unless absorption takes place, as has been outlined, it will be NECESSARY to use more of a heavier course. 5451-6 /Cataracts/

****

5. (Q) Is there anything that can be done for my eyes, so that I won't have to wear glasses?
(A) The correction of the conditions in the cervical, and the treatment with the *Violet Ray* will materially aid these. Especially will the body use, after the first three to five treatments - or after the

2nd or third week - the *Violet Ray* applicator for the eyes, but not treating the eyes longer than one minute. Well, too, while these are being given - that is, during the same period, of evenings when the body rests, to place scraped Irish potato, with which is mixed almost equal parts of plain chalk - place this over the eyes, bind on, and of mornings cleanse the eyes with that of a weak solution of an antiseptic, like boracic acid.   5571-1/Eyes: Spine: Subluxations/

****

11. We would also find that the application of the *Violet Ray* to the upper dorsal and the cervical area will relieve the tension at times to the eye, as well as to the heart's circulation. Such treatments we would not take too great a period at a time, especially until there had been sufficient lapse of time or sufficient activity with the equalizing conditions in the low form of the vibrations from the Radio-Active forces. The applications would be made as the body is ready to retire, or when there come those periods of overanxiety from the strain from any of the activities in the system. From ten to twelve minutes would be sufficient each time, making the application three to four times a week - the hand *Violet Ray* machine.   403-2Circulation: Incoordination/

****

7. For the condition of the eye, apply the *Violet Ray*, eye applicator. Do this about twice a week. Follow with placing a scraped Irish potato poultice over the eye to cleanse same. Use any good antiseptic to wash out. This should prevent accumulation, and clear the eye of the shadow of the cataract, which is tending to form there, but the eliminations will have to be set up much better.   326-15/Cataracts/

VARIOUS ANODE APPLICATORS OR ATTACHMENTS REFERRED TO IN THE CAYCE READINGS

BULB APPLICATOR

4. We would add a very little of the electrical forces for the body, though, in the present. To do this will prevent the central nervous system batteries from running down. This should be used in the form of the *Violet Ray* - hand machine, bulb applicator; but don't give it more than half a minute, and don't give it about the head. Give it across the sacral and the back, at the diaphragm, and this not more than half to three-quarters of a minute - just before retiring. It'll pick the body up! 2528-4/Circulation: Cold/

****

13. Also we would have the stimulating vibrations from the Violet Ray (with the flat bulb or the large bulb) applied each evening just before retiring, for three to four minutes; especially across the

shoulders, over the back of the neck, around the face, down and across the diaphragm area. **This will STIMULATE the circulation and be activative with those forces that are taken internally through the tonic as well as working with the diets of the body.** 412-8/Eliminations: Incoordination/

****

6. Also take once each day, preferably in the morning, the vibrations over the throat, head and lower portion of spine and abdomen of the *Violet Ray*, with the bulb applicator; not with the direct or too long a ray, nor over the chest, but over the upper bronchials, throat, thyroids, head, back from the first cervical to the toes.
 7. Do this. We will find we will assist this vibration to keep in the equilibrium necessary. Do not give this vibration for more than five minutes at one time to the body. 304-4/Asthma/

38. But after they have been begun, or after the first fifteen days, then we would begin to apply the PLAIN *Violet Ray* each evening when ready to retire; using the bulb applicator. This would be given not at high rate or speed but at that so the body will respond to same. In the application begin at the base of the head (the body lying prone), massage it gently in a ROTARY motion (back and forth across the spine, see?) across shoulders, across the abdominal area (from the back), across the lower sacral area and to the end of the spine; then along the sciatic nerves to the heels, then along the arm to the wrist; and then on the FRONTAL portion of the body, gently across the diaphragm, the liver and the caecum area on the right portion, you see. In all take at least eight to ten minutes for such a treatment. Each day CLEANSE the BULB or the anode. 1044-1 /Flu: After Effects/

****

The authors have used several methods to clean the bulb. One is to use a solution of baking soda and water to cleanse the glass area that comes in contact with the skin. The second is to use soap and water to remove the film that will collect on the glass area that contacts the skin.

ROD APPLICATOR

Note: The rod applicator recommended in the following reading is to be made of metal. In the other readings listed, this is not specified. A glass rod applicator is available, however, and one must take special care if using it in the manner described in the following reading as the applicator will be more fragile.

****

14. Also we would give the low electrical vibrations of the *Violet Ray* (hand machine), but not with the bulb applicator. Rather use the *metal rod applicator* that is held in the hand, or it may be held in the hand one time and the next time the foot placed upon it - with the rod lying upon a piece of glass, you see - the bare foot placed on it. Take this for at least a minute and a half, or for two to three minutes, each evening - preferably just before ready to retire; one evening holding it in the hand, the next evening setting the foot upon it - opposite extremity, you see; continuing to alternate in this manner. 2058-2 /Colds: Debilitation/Toxemia/

****

5. The electrical forces would best be taken with the *Violet Ray*. The body can best do this itself. Obtain a medium- priced *Violet Ray* (hand machine). Do not turn on full force, and use ONLY the rod applicator, or the applicator that is held in the hand. But use this also on the feet; that is: Place the connection or anode or applicator on a piece of glass (just a pane of glass put on the floor, you see), and then place the foot on same. The next day take it in the opposite hand, the next the opposite foot, the next the opposite hand. Do not take this, though, for more than a minute at a time for the first week or ten days. Afterwards it may be increased to a minute and a half or two minutes, as the general condition of the circulation and the general toxic forces improve. Be mindful to take these as indicated for the body, in the present; not the bulb applicator or as of the hand electricity, but the high vibrations that go directly to the body - though very mild at first, and take these just before retiring of night. One day hold the applicator in the right hand, the next day put the left foot on it (with the applicator placed on glass first, you see), the next day hold the right foot on it, the next day hold it in the left hand, see? and so on.

261-35/Toxemia/

****

28. Begin immediately when these osteopathic treatments are begun, with the use of the *Violet Ray*. These vibrations may be taken at home, or just before retiring. A small portion of same should be applied about the head, the ear, the brachial center, the dorsal center, the lumbar center, and then across the diaphragm area. Then for three to five minutes just take the plain applicator (rod applicator) and hold in the hand.   1164-1/Assimilations: Eliminations: Incoordination/

****

11. And we would CONTROL same by the massages and the low electrical forces that may be had by the hand *Violet Ray*.

12. And rather than making most of these applications of the *Violet Ray* with the bulb appliance, we would use the rod that charges the whole system - and especially to the lower limbs.

1137-1/Violet Ray: Rheumatism/

****

16. After such a vibrator treatment REST for a period of fifteen to twenty minutes. THEN use the Hand Machine *Violet Ray*, but preferably with the applicator that is held in the hand - that is, the rod applicator. Take it a minute in the beginning, and gradually increase it to a minute and a quarter and then after a few days to a minute and a half; then after another five to ten days take it for two minutes. For the first eight to ten to fifteen treatments, hold the applicator in the right hand. Then after that it may be alternated about the body; that is, one day it would be held in the right hand, the next day it would be laid on a piece of glass on the floor and the left foot set upon it; the next day it would be held in the left hand, the next day the right foot would be set on it; and so on around the body - but for the first ten to fifteen treatments, as indicated, use only in the right hand.

1572-1/Possession/

****

13. After this has been taken once or twice, we would also begin with the use of the *Violet Ray*. The greater portion of this, or the better way to take same, would be through the extremities; not with the bulb applicator but with the hand or rod applicator, see? This would just be held in the hand (or under the foot) to, in a manner, recharge the body. Do not take too much at a time. First hold it in the left hand, for half a minute. Then, removing the shoe and sock on the right foot, set the applicator on glass and lay the right foot on same for half a minute. The next time (and this should be taken at least three times a week) hold in the right hand first, for half a minute, then put the left foot on same for half a minute, in the same way and manner. Not more than a minute, then, for the whole treatment, see? 984-3/Circulation:Incoordination/

****

20. After there have been three or four of the osteopathic adjustments, begin then also (not before) with the *Violet Ray*, hand machine - but not the bulb applicator. Rather use the rod applicator that may be held in the hand, or the foot placed upon same. It would be better if it is taken one time in the hand, the next time laying the rod anode upon a piece of glass and placing the bare foot on same. Use this for two minutes each day (when it is begun) for five days, leave off five days, and then take again for five days, and so on. 2536-1/Osteopathy: Relaxation/

****

COMB APPLICATOR

20. (Q) Please itemize treatment for scalp and shampoo.
(A) The better treatment for the scalp would be the *Violet Ray*, using the comb applicator that will stimulate the scalp itself. But unless these corrections are made, the circulation to the scalp will not be proper, see? 494-1/Skin: Scalp: Circulation/

****

Stimulation of the scalp and the area of the thyroid system are indicated to help prevent the hair from graying.

52. (Q) What causes the hair to fade? How may life be restored?
(A) Use the scalp applicator of the *Violet Ray* occasionally. The general stimulation to the activities of the glandular system, with these applications indicated, will aid much. For remember, all of these - the cuticle, the skin, the hair, the activities of all of these natures - arise from the functionings of the thyroid system, see? 1563-1/Glands: Thyroid: Hair/

****

For coordinating the superficial and deep circulation, use the Violet Ray as well as to stimulate growth of hair on the scalp.

34. (Q) What treatment should be used for the scalp?
(A) The electrical treatment with the *Violet Ray* for this particular body, we find, would be the MOST beneficial.
35. (Q) Will this prevent the hair falling out?
(A) As indicated, there have been those tendencies for the superficial and the deeper circulations to be disturbed. They are breaking away, they are not coordinating. A stimulation to any portion of the body for greater activity, by not too much but as using the comb of such a hand *Violet Ray* machine through the hair and head, will make for such stimulation as to make more growth of the hair and also a better growth of the hair.   1120-2/Violet Ray: Hair

****

15. (Q) What causes gray hair, and how can it be prevented?
(A) This arises from many, many causes, - but it is a general condition of the stimulation to the scalp pores or of the hair itself. It may be worry, it may come from anxiety, it may come from fear or fright, or from - as indicated - lack of elements in the superficial circulation. In the type of circulation as indicated, as we find here, - when the body uses the *Violet Ray*, use also occasionally - not every time, but occasionally - the scalp applicator, or that which works like a rake through same, see?   1947-4/ Incoordination: Color Restorer/

SOME DON'TS FOR THE VIOLET RAY USER

21. Abstain from ANY intoxicating drinks of ANY kind! This means even beer, too! Too much of these, with the electrical forces (if they are to be taken), will be DETRIMENTAL to the better conditions of the body.
22. Electricity and alcohol don't work together! It burns tissue, and is not good for ANYBODY!
323-1/Alcohol & Electricity: General/

****

12. (Q) Should *Violet Ray* be used; how and when?
(A) We would not use the Violet Ray until less of the disturbances are indicated through the alimentary canal; and then it would be used principally over the lower portions of the body, - from the 9th dorsal down, and extending along the limbs, - it would be most helpful.   313-20/Colon: Engorgement/

****

325-60 Warns: Do not use the Violet Ray, Ultra-Violet Ray or Ash within 3 to 4 days of X-ray Treatments.

15. (Q) **If X-Ray flashes are given, what should be done about the Ash, and the present lamp that she uses daily?**
(A) **We have indicated that these would not be given at the same time; but three to four days after the X-Ray treatments use the *Violet Ray* hand machine, NOT the ultra-Violet Ray, following the small doses of Ash taken.**   325-60/Cancer: Breast/

****

22. (Q) **Considering present treatments, how often should hand massage *Violet Ray* be given, at home?**
(A) **As indicated, if the X-Ray flashes are used we would not use the *Violet Ray*; especially when they are given every day! We have given this again and again! The hand massage, as indicated, would be well - gently - to induce sleep, in the evenings. But leave off the machine while the X-Ray treatments are being given!** 325-64/Cancer: Breast/

***Note**: The Violet Ray Hand Machine, #504 and #555, can only be used for a maximum of 10 minutes per session. The unit must then be cooled.*

ATTITUDE

***Note**: Cayce states throughout the readings that the Mind is the Builder. Visualization is one way of training the mind to impart its wisdom to the body. Visualization exists in a no-time framework, the realm of the mind. Allow the body to catch up to the message of the vision for its framework exists in time.*

8. At times we find these conditions get on the nerves of the body, as it were, and the body ceases to care to put up the resistance, feeling as if there is no use. This should be dismissed, for the body should acquire and gain, and set before self, that all building and replenishing for a physical body is from within, and must be constructed by the mind of the entity; for MIND is the BUILDER; for each cell in the atomic force of the body is as a world of its own, and each one - each cell - being in perfect unison, may build to that necessary to reconstruct the forces of the body in all its needs, and in this body, as given, there is then necessary to add that vibration to that being administered, that would give this incentive, necessary in rest, necessary in blood building, necessary in the cellular forces of the body, for these to coordinate the more properly, would we bring the better physical forces to the body. 93-1/Mind: The Builder/

*****

33. (Q) Please give body a mental suggestion which will help her to maintain her desire to get well, and have confidence again in herself.
(A) Keep that mental attitude of helpfulness, usefulness to those that the body may influence in its activity. And leave the results of ALL conditions in the hands of Him that giveth life, light and immortality. Let THOSE be as thy axioms: *"Let the words of my mouth, the meditations of my heart, be acceptable in Thy sight, my Lord, and my Redeemer."*   325-61/Cancer: Breast/ or Meditation:Affirmation/

****

2. Do that. Be persistent, be consistent, and with each application, with each adjustment, with each application of the Violet Ray, of all mechanical forces as is given in the body, let the mental forces create, give, build, magnify in this physical body the ability of the healing forces to come to this body.
4602-2/Locomotion: Impaired/

****

13. (Q) Any other advice?
(A) Keep that same helpful and hopeful mental attitude towards the using of the vision, and the mental and spiritual self, for helpfulness to others.   1861-4/Soul Development/

****

4. First there needs to be much changed in the general physical and mental attitude of the body. So long as the body holds to the attitude that the world and everything in it is against the activities of the body and the thought of its better welfare, so long as the body is continuing to feel sorry for itself, it will continue to have greater and greater disturbances through the physical forces of the body.
3574-1/Attitudes & Emotions: Self-Pity/

25. Let THIS be the attitude of the body: Not as rote, but that there may be awakened in every atom of the physical forces of the body the DIVINE within.   679-1/Eyes: Retina/

****

3. First, do not dwell mentally so much upon the conditions of the body by magnifying them in thine own experience. Rather choose a manner of activity and live, act, be in mental and physical, the expectancy of gaining results. That is the first attitude.
4. But to continue to dwell upon those conditions as to physical that disturb the body tends to magnify them and necessarily the body has to meet them.
5. If we magnify the surroundings and make for those expressions of resentment in this or that way or manner, there is builded in the mental attitude those resistances to be met in the mental and physical forces of the body.
6. If there is the continual feeling sorry for self, condemning someone else or looking toward the idea that there is not this or that experience in self as for someone else, then these - too - in the attitude - bring aggravations to the general system.
1195-2/Cancer: Tendencies/

****

CHAPTER THREE

The Scientific Healing Method

Instruction Booklet found in the Violet Rays manufactured in the early to mid 1900's.

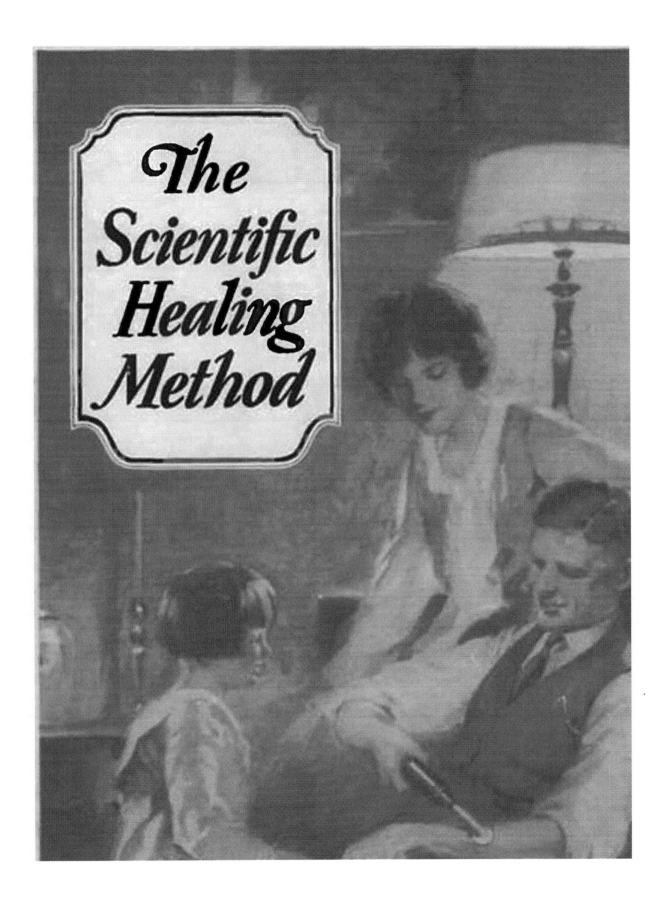

The Scientific Healing Method

Electricity and Health

AS scientists penetrate deeper and deeper into the mysteries of life, their discoveries tend to prove that the fudamental basis of life is to be found in electrical energy manifested by the Electron.

What An Electron Is

The Electron — the basis of all fundamental matter, both living and inanimate—may be defined as the smallest conceivable amount of electricity. For example study of chemistry shows us that pure water is made up of the two elements, hydrogen and oxygen, combined in a ratio of 2 atoms of hydrogen to each 1 atom of oxygen. Well, each infinitesimal atom contains a number of electrical particles—called Electrons.

In the human body and plants as well, we know that the various parts and organs are made up of thousands and thousands of minute cells and if all matter contains electrons, as is the accepted belief— the fundamental processes of the cell are electrical. This theory is not in conflict with the chemical theory—as chemistry defines the complex formations and arrangements of the various atoms— the electron as a constituent of the atom offers the logical explanation for chemical actions.

Function of Body is Electrical

The functions of the human body are basically electrical in their nature. Life itself can be said to depend primarily upon the functioning of the electron.

High Frequency Current

During the last decade we have become more familar with a special kind of current. This is High Frequency current which oscillates back and forth with great rapidity giving rise to distinctive and interesting phenomena. This type of current is the basis for radio and is called Radio Frequency.

Even before the day of radio, High Frequency currents were known and a number of medical and scientific men had carried on experiments to determine their effects on the human body, it being logical to assume that since the fundamental processes of life are electrical, High Frequency current might be used to stimulate the body cells and accelerate their functioning.

The discoveries of these scientists in their application of High Frequency currents to the human system established the answers to five perplexing questions:
1. High frequency currents increase metabolism—the building up of cell structure by oxidation and natural nutrition.
2. It stimulates and increases the flow of blood to given areas. This is called Hyperemia.
3. It increases secretion.
4. Stimulates and soothes body areas according to length of application.
5. Renders more complete the elimination of waste products.

What Is Metabolism?

Stated briefly METABOLISM consists of the changes continually going on in living cells by which energy is provided for growth of these cells (see illustration No. 1).

The human body—its tissue, muscles, bones, nerves, hair, nails, etc.,—is like a honey comb of millions of microscopic cells and though these various cell groups differ in their structure and function—they all are alive and dependent on electrical activity. For these cells to live and function healthfully they must (a) absorb sufficient oxygen to feed the cell and keep it vigorous, (b) chemically combine and use the oxygen absorbed. (c) throw off the waste products created by this combustion. Normal cell activity with all these processes functioning properly, is Health.

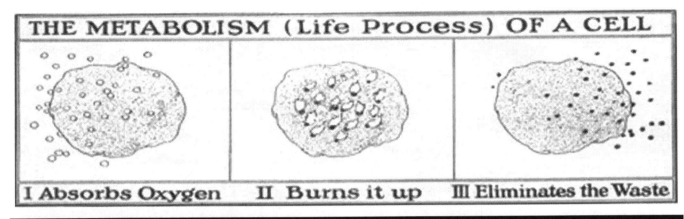

THE METABOLISM (Life Process) OF A CELL

I Absorbs Oxygen   II Burns it up   III Eliminates the Waste

Illustration No. 1

If any one of these three functions of normal cell action ceases or even is hindered, it throws out of balance the well being (health) of the cell as a whole. If all these functions stop, the cell dies.

Life Process of a cell. The great majority of constitutional ailments may be traced to the failure of the functioning of certain cells to absorb sufficient oxygen, combine it for combustion properly, or completely eliminate the waste. In rheumatism, the failure is in the proper elimination of the waste clogging up in the tissues and causing painful swellings.

High Frequency Current Penetrates and Reaches Ailing Cells

High Frequency currents have the power to penetrate the ailing cells stimulating and causing them to function normally, thereby carrying out the Life Process or Metabolism.

High Frequency Application For Home Use Now at Low Cost

The application of High Frequency current formerly required an elaborate and expensive apparatus. Today this is no longer necessary. A very compact and efficient generator may be had at such a price as to be within reach of everybody. All the necessary electrical apparatus is combined in the bakelite housing and the entire unit may be held very conveniently in the hand.

(See Illustration No. 2)

The High Frequency current is applied by means of the glass vacuum attachment, commonly called the electrode. These electrodes act in the same manner as a fine spray nozzle attached to a high pressure stream of water. The electrode breaks up the concentrated high pressure stream of electricity into a gentle and soothing mist of revitalizing energy.

There is no sensation or shock in connection with the treatment. The electrode is simply inserted into the instrument and lightly rubbed over the afflicted ailing member. There is a sensation of heat and stimulation after a few minutes. You will enjoy its mild stimulation.

Many Ailments Treated Successfully with Violet Rays

The following list of ailments may seem quite large for one form of treatment to cover but when the cause of all pain is analyzed it is quite natural that

Stimulates Circulation

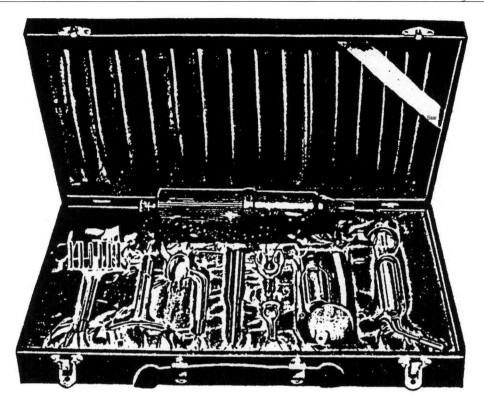

Illustration **No. 2**

the application of High Frequency currents should be beneficial in these various ailments.

High Frequency treatment is primarily for the relief of pain without the
use of drugs. **It is a home remedy and
is not intended to replace the Physician
in his rightful place.** (See illustration
No. 3)

1. ABSCESSES:

All circumscribed collections of pus
are termed abscesses, and are usually
the result of inflamed connective tissue.
**Pain is relieved, the cause removed and
suppuration arrested by three or four
applications of medium to strong current 3 to 5 minutes once or twice a day.**

2. ARTHRITIS:

Arthritis is a disease of a wide classi-
fication. Some years ago it was generally called rheumatism, without any attempt at differentiation. There are many
forms of arthritis, each one somewhere
similar in symptons and all are characterized by pain of more or less difference.
Among the more common forms is
Acute Rheumatic Arthritis. Certain fea-
tures being a sudden onset of pain and
swelling in the joints with a certain degree of redness. After a day or two it
seems to travel from one joint to another.

**Rheumatic Arthritis is frequently chro-
nic and requires patience and constant
treatment over a more or less long
period of time. The High Frequency
current should be applied twice daily
over the affected parts, using the No. 1
electrode.** The splendid success secured
with the aid of High Frequency treatment in this ailment has been most
gratifying. The promptness with which
pain is relieved places this form of treatment in the foremost ranks.

Produces   Muscular   And   Cellular   Massage

38. WRITER'S CRAMP:

Decided benefit is obtained by one treatment a day using medium current from shoulder to finger tips five minutes.

39. WRINKLES:

Neither medical nor mechanical science has or will produce any process by which the marks of time may be wholly erased. The abnormal contraction of some muscles, the relaxation of others, and the thickening of tissue are fixations of the years that no human hand can undo. The suggestion of this treatment as an agency for modifying these hand-marks of time is wholly predicated upon its action and results already stated: its penetrating processes in breaking down congested tissue, effecting elimination of toxic deposits, relaxation of muscular tension, increased circulation and increased local nutrition. These do aid in smoothing the wrinkles by restoring muscular balance.

Apply medium current to face, neck, throat, arms and hands, moving Electrode slowly and in a rotary motion. Daily treatments of about seven minutes should be taken. To assure an evening of that mental and physical vivacity which every woman so greatly admires, no stimulant is so positively, so naturally and so permanently effective as a few minutes with the High Frequency. For the "Ionic massage", hold Electrode No. 1

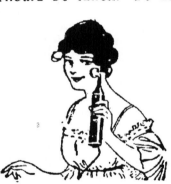

Illustration No. 6

in hand and apply strong current, four minutes. Treat spine, base of brain, temples and forehead with medium current four minutes. Apply medium to strong current to cheeks, holding Electrode in loose contact, two minutes.

High Frequency Electrodes

Although the High Frequency Outfits as made up are equipped with a selection of the most important electrodes or applicators, you may make it still more complete and greatly increase the satisfaction and comfort of its use by getting additional electrodes, which, as you will see from the illustrations and descriptions, are especially made for the treatment of a long list of ailments. The Tips are uniform so that all electrodes will fit the standard generator handle you may have. Write your nearest store for prices on any of the electrodes in which you are interested.

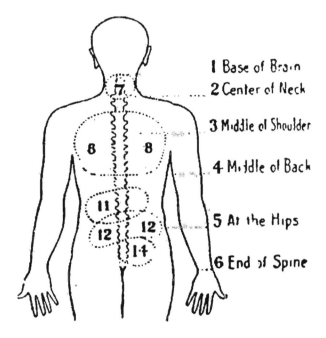

1 Base of Brain
2 Center of Neck
3 Middle of Shoulder
4 Middle of Back
5 At the Hips
6 End of Spine

S t i m u l a t e s   C i r c u l a t i o n

GOUTY ARTHRITIS:

This form of arthritis is generally one of faulty metabolism. Apply High Frequency current to both feet and limbs, using the No. 1 electrode. Also treat over liver, area No. 11, for a period of five minutes.

3. ASTHMA:

Apply medium to strong current five to seven minutes over throat and chest or until muscular spasm is relieved. Daily Ozone inhalations should be taken.

4. BACKACHE:

Strong current five minutes over affected area gives relief.

5. BOILS, CARBUNCLES, FELONS:

Carbuncles being more deeply seated should be treated with stronger currents otherwise follow directions for Abscesses.

6. BRAIN AND NERVE FATIGUE:

Medium current over temples, forehead and base of brain five minutes and over entire spine six minutes daily. This treatment with five minutes Ozone inhalations has been likened by a physician to "a day in the Alps".

7. BRONCHITIS:

The following is from a clinical report: "In cases of bronchitis, asthma and pneumonia, applications of high frequency currents to chest and throat procure long lasting results". Apply with strong current five to seven minutes. Ozone inhalations are very beneficial.

8. BUNIONS:

Three to five minutes medium to strong current through sock or stocking brings instant relief of pain. Daily treatments usually give permanent relief.

9. COLD HANDS AND FEET:

To restore circulation, which is the object, apply strong current to each member three minutes daily.

10. CHAPPED HANDS AND FACE:

Application of mild current three to five minutes at night brings gratifying relief.

11. CHILBLAINS:

Apply with strong current four to six minutes daily.

12. CATARRH (Nasal):

Apply over nose, cheek bones, temples and forehead five minutes with medium current. Ozone inhalations five minutes. If relief is not had use Nasal Electrode No. 11 inserted deeply and apply medium current in each nostril three minutes.

13. CONSTIPATION:

This troublesome condition, probably the one way most travelled to serious complications and diseases, has a number of causes, the most common and the one always present in chronic constipation is faulty circulation, malnutrition and interrupted elimination in the intestinal capillary field with consequent impaired functional activity of the parastaltic and abdominal muscles.

After months, perhaps years of recourse to cathartics, which excite but do not stimulate these functional activities, with whatever aid, nature cannot restore normal conditions over-night; and High Frequency offers no "miracle-cures". It is scarcely necessary to repeat its processes, — its penetrating molecular or "ionic massage" carrying heat and chemical action to the intestinal capillary field, affecting elimination of congested tissue and increased circulation of nutrient blood. But even with this aid, the patient must also give nature a hand. Attention must be given to diet, not dieting, but a reasonable consumption of foods rich in water in cellulose or fibre, plenty of water, and regular habit of daily evacuation. One-half teaspoonful of salt dissolved in one pint of hot water and taken thirty minutes before breakfast will aid.

Begin with two treatments a day. As improvement is established, once a day, then twice a week until normal condition returns. Apply medium current over about one foot of middle spine five minutes and strong current over entire stomach and abdominal area six minutes. If relief is not apparent within a few days use Rectal Electrode No. 14 once a day. Insert deeply and apply medium current five minutes.

14. CORNS AND CALLUSES:

These "little pain-devils" as they are sometimes called with good provocation, present a very concrete example of nerve-pressure and its results. Prompt relief of pain is had by applying current from edge of Electrode No. 1 or point of Rectal Electrode No. 14. To remove, use cautery Electrode No. 20, applying current once a week for about thirty seconds on callused tissue.

15. CRAMP:

Strong current relieves the muscular spasm and restores circulation. High Frequency current is one of the most effective means of relieving this painful condition. The compacted muscles are almost instantly relieved under the soothing action of the current.

16. DANDRUFF, FALLING HAIR, ITCHING SCALP:

Bacterial infection and impaired circualtion are the usual sources of these troubles. Daily treatments with Comb Electrode No. 3 held in close but gentle contact with scalp, applying mild current five minutes, quickly relieves itching and dandruff, stops falling hair and in many cases restores growth of hair. High Frequency Violet Ray treatments are accepted as standard by nearly all Beauty Specialists and Beauticians throughout the country. It is one of the most effective means of stimulating the circulation of the blood, thus supplying the proper nutrition to the roots of the hair. The tingling and refreshing after sensation is most pleasant and stimulating.

17. DEAFNESS:

Most frequently deafness is the result of a catarrhal condition with inflammation of and consequent congestion and closure of the eustachian tube. Due to the character of these currents, their penetrating massage carrying Ozone, probably the most corrective agency for catarrh, effecting a breaking down and elimination of congested tissue and restoring local circulation. Partial deafness responds in most cases with very gratifying results. Insert Electrode No. 11 deeply in the ear and apply mild current three to five minutes. Follow with Electrode No. 1 around ear five minutes, medium current. A quick relief of earache.

18. DYSPEPSIA:

Where atonic, catarrhal and nervous conditions are the cause, these treatments are always highly beneficial. Treat over middle spine with medium current five minutes and over stomach with stronger current five minutes daily.

19. ECZEMA:

Itching is immediately relieved by applying short sparks from edge of Electrode. Cover affected area with rather strong current three to five minutes according to size of affected area, and repeat treatment as often as itching returns.

20. ENLARGED PROSTATE:

The term of hypertrophy of the prostate is applied to that form of enlargement of the gland which takes place after middle life, sometimes before the fiftieth year, and more frequently after the age of sixty, developing slowly and without inflammatory symptoms. The cause of the condition is unknown. The affection is first accompanied by an increased frequency of urination, particularly at night, lessened force of the stream, inability to entirely empty the bladder and consequent retention of

Stimulates Circulation

urine. Cystitic and kidney disease are likely to follow this condition.

Acute Prostatic may result from exposure to cold and wet, from wound or external injury and from disease. It is characterized by a sensation of heat or weight in the rectum and by pain and very frequent and unavailing effort to evacuate the bladder or bowels.

Enlargement of the prostate is not growth. While as stated by this authority no cause is known for the functional failure, enlargement is due to impaired circulation and thickening and hardening the gland tissue. Thus ensues an ever tightening pressure upon the uretha and gradual lessening of the urinary flow. During this progressive enlargement patients often suffer from backache, headache, neuritis, sciatica and other pains without suspecting the real cause of their discomforts. The most serious consequences follow that condition when the enlargement becomes so great as to form a cone within the bladder, thus making it impossible to entirely empty the bladder. The result is that this residual urine sets up inflammation of the bladder and invites other serious consequences.

Other than surgical removal a reduction of the enlargement is the only remedy. The processes by which High Frequency Violet Ray currents effect this relief are the same as in every other condition of congested tissue. By use of the insulated prostate electrode, the currents are applied undiffused direct to the prostate gland, thus generating heat, chemical action and effecting a tissue massage of one million oscillations a second.

Treatment is easily and conveniently administered by one's self. Lying upon the back with knees drawn up and with Special Prostate Electrode No. 9-A in instrument turned to the side under right knee. Insert slowly, giving the rectal muscles time to relax. With ring against the anus the electrode is in position to apply current direct to prostate gland. Treat five to seven minutes with current strong enough to effect perceptible but not uncomfortable heat. Then apply strong current over bladder five minutes with electrode No. 1. Begin with two treatments a day then once a day, twice a week, once a week, once a month, or as required.

21. FACE PIMPLES AND BLACK-HEADS:

Apply medium current once a day for four minutes. Where postules are large turn edge of Electrode to effect short sparks. Avoid constipation.

22. GOITRE:

A morbid enlargement of the thyroid gland from unknown cause. The object, like that of enlarged prostate is to effect elimination or absorption of the congested tissue. While not as prompt nor so universally positive as with the prostate, many physicians report highly satisfactory results. In many cases enlargement is arrested, in many marked reduction is effected and apparent permanent relief obtained. Treat entire surface of goitre six minutes with strong current once a day.

23. GOUT:

A constitutional disease characterized by excess of uric acid or alkaline urates. The main object is elimination of these toxic causes. Treat with strong current over liver, kidneys and bladder, giving four minutes to each, then over seat of pain with mild current three or four minutes.

24. HAY FEVER:

Severity of attack is modified by five minutes application of medium current to nose and forehead and five minutes Ozone inhalations twice a day.

Produces   Muscular   And   Cellular   Massage

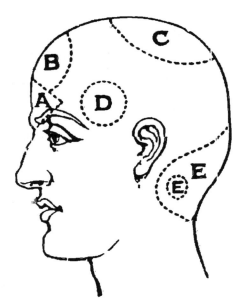

Illustration No. 4

Showing areas where headaches occur.

25. HEADACHES:

A headache is the sympton of some constitutional disorder; it is not a distinct disease. Illustration No. 4 shows you how you can tell the cause of any headache. It will be useful in suggesting the probable line of treatment.

Headaches at A or B are congestive of frontal and may be relieved by passing the Electrode No. 1 back and forth over the seat of pain. At A they may come from errors in refraction, frontal sinus disease or nasal disease. Stomach diseases also frequently cause pain at A. Constipation, A-B. Decay of front teeth, A-B. Anemia, endometritis, bladder disease, C. Middle ear disease, throat disease, eye disease, decayed teeth, D-E. Womb disease, spinal irritation, nervousness, E. Ovarion reflex pains usually at C and E. Neurasthenic headaches involve the back of the neck.

26. INSOMNIA:

Sleeplessness is caused by one or more of three conditions: congested brain cells, digestive disturbances or nervousness. It is unnecessary to restate the processes by which this treatment relieves these conditions. Before retiring take "ionic massage" five minutes, treat with mild current over spine and base of brain four minutes, and with stronger current over stomach five minutes. Ozone inhalations are of value.

27. LUMBAGO:

This severe paroxysmal form of muscular rheumatism of the loins and their tendinous attachments responds most gratifyingly to strong currents. Patient should move in different positions and treat painful locations as movement developes them. Treat through cloth the thickness of turkish towel. Five to seven minutes may be required to bring relief.

28. NEURALGIA:

Apply to local area of pain five minutes. If not relieved apply medium current to upper spine and base of brain five minutes and strong current to stomach four minutes.

29. NEURITIS:

Not frequently first treatments accentuate the pain. Continued, they invariably bring relief. This is an inflammation of the nerve-trunks and it is only necessary to reflect upon the processes of these currents to understand how and why nature restores itself by their aid. Treatment should be by mild current and from three to five minutes along the course of the nerves. A clinical authority says: "There is no doubt that the D'Arsonval currents can relieve pain and procure sleep after all other methods have failed.

30. PARALYSIS:

Medically defined as "Loss of power of voluntary motion resulting from

58

structural change of brain, spinal cord, nerves or muscles." Where the cause is cerebral, little may be expected. If the result of spinal, nerve or muscle derangement good results are had. INFANTILE PARALYSIS, usually a spinal affection is gratifyingly responsive. Treatment is the same in both cases. Strong current should be used daily, five minutes over spine and five to seven minutes over affected members. Twice a week treat through cloth thick enough to affect a counterirritant sufficient to redden the skin.

31. RHEUMATISM:

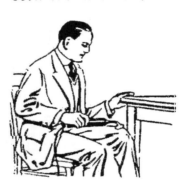

Illustration No. 5

One of the most painful and most difficult diseases to relieve. No drug has been found that is more than palliative. Thermal baths are probably the most satisfactory treatment. But for those millions who are unable to avail themselves of that treatment **High Frequency** offers a very excellent and effective treatment agent. What is desired — what must be effected to obtain relief— is the elimination of toxic deposits in tissue and joints. If the condition is muscular treat as for lumbago; if of joints treat as for Arthritis.

32. RINGWORM:

Ringworm is a contagious vegetable or fungus parasitic infection attacking the scalp, bearded portions of the face and other parts of the body and is one of the most difficult skin diseases to control. Apply strong current three to five minutes according to size of affected area and where postules are present turn edge of Electrode to effect sparks. Daily treatments for a week or ten days effect permanent relief.

33. SCIATICA:

The sciatic nerve is very deeply imbedded under the large outer muscles of the leg. Its invariable response to these currents is the result of their unvarying penetrating oscillating, heat-creating and chemical producing processes direct upon the nerve itself. Apply strong currents to painful locality and along the course of the nerve five to seven minutes.

34. SINUS TROUBLE:

While the suggestion is not made that this painful and difficult condition will be altogether relieved, modifications of pain and increased comfort is affected by the application of medium currents over affected area five minutes twice a day. Once a day, with Electrode placed on one side of forehead, have an assistant draw the current through the sinus by placing the hand on opposite side of forehead. Take daily Ozone Inhalations.

35. SPRAINS:

Use strong current five to seven minutes with Electrode to light contact and repeat treatment as condition requires.

36. TIRED ACHING FEET:

Five minutes strong current to each foot effects gratifying relief.

37. WARTS:

These disfiguring growths may be safely, painlessly and quickly removed by the use of Cautery Electrode No. 20. Apply mild current over growth (taking care to keep off healthy surface) until a whitish-brown color appears. Metal point should be held so as to effect short sparks or stream of florescene. Repeat in a week if growth hasnot dropped off.

R e l i e v e s   A c h e s   A n d   P a i n s

ILLUSTRATION NO. 3

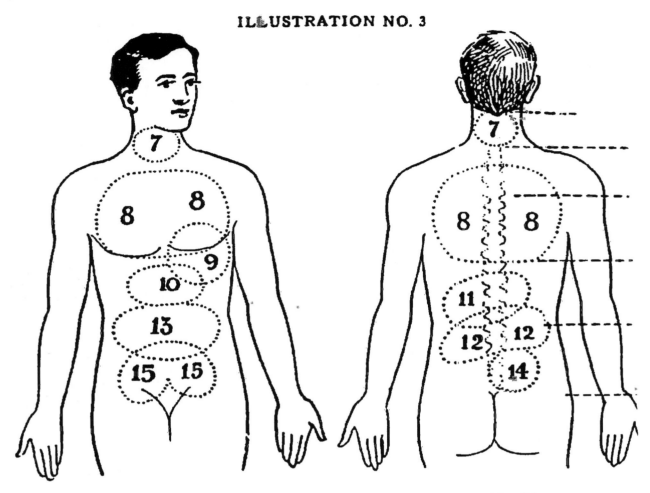

1. Base of Brain.
2. Center of Neck.
3. Middle of Shoulder.
4. Middle of Back.
5. Hips.
6. End of Spine.
7. Neck and Throat.
8. Lungs.
9. Heart.
10. Stomach.
11. Liver.
12. Kidneys.
13. Bowels.
14. Spleen.
15. Loins.

Septic Arthritis— This form does not affect one joint after another as in Rheumatic Arthritis. The trouble is due to a source of infection. the toxins being carried by the blood stream and deposited at some joint. causing pain and swelling. Abscesses of one form or another, particularly of the teeth. are the main contributing factors of this condition. Obviously the treatment consists of relieving the infection first. This should be done before using the High Frequency current. Frequently the joint or limb is left in an impaired condition after an attack and excellent results in restoring it to normal after the focus of infection is cleared up by the use of the High Frequency current using applicator No. 1 over the affected area. Use the No. 1 electrode for a period of five to ten minutes twice daily over the affected and painful parts.

Soothes Tired Nerves

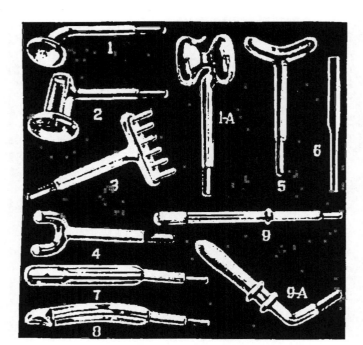

Spinal action, use the Metal Spinal Electrode No. 30.

No. 5 Throat Electrode.—designed so as to fit over the neck. Very excellent results have been accomplished with this electrode in Goitre, Tonsilitis, Double Chin and Bronchial Troubles. Any excessive formation is eliminated.

No. 6 Metal Electrode.—This delivers a strong current and is excellent for general tonic and where constitutional effects are desired.

When held by the patient there is no muscular contraction, merely a sense of glowing warmth permeating the entire body. The current can also be drawn to any part of the body by using No. 1 electrode or the fingers of the operator.

Insulated Electrodes

The advantage of insulated electrodes is the fact that the current may be introduced without loss into the orifice of the body. In the plain electrodes much of the current is drawn off at the first point of contact.

No. 7 Special Vaginal Electrode with perforations so that Ozone may be generated within the vagina. Used for ovaritis, leucorrhea etc.

No. 8 Vaginal Electrode without perforations.

No. 9A Prostatic Electrode—Specially designed and constructed for the treatment of prostatitis. Length is just right to reach prostate gland. Insulated to the tip and shaped for most comfortable position.

No. 1 General Electrode.—Used for facial and body treatments, and for any surface application. This electrode is constructed in such a manner as to prevent the current from heating, which is likely to cause it to break. For this reason it will outlast other makes.

No. 2 Condenser Electrode.—As the name implies, it condenses the current, and produces a strong even flow; also generating electrical heat which is very desirable in deep seated cases.
Used for Rheumatism, Lumbago, Neuritis, Neurasthenia, Skin Disease, etc. This Electrode can be used in place of the No. 1 or No. 6, where stronger spark is desired.

No. 3 Comb-Rake Electrode.—Used for all scalp treatments; Falling Hair, Dandruff, Gray Hair and for stimulating the hair roots and cells.

No. 4 Spinal Electrode.—For all spinal treatments. Arranged so that it fits over both sides of the vertibrae. For Reflex

Produces Muscular And Cellular Massage

It will more than pay for itself within six months in the average household. The life of the generator is indefinite.

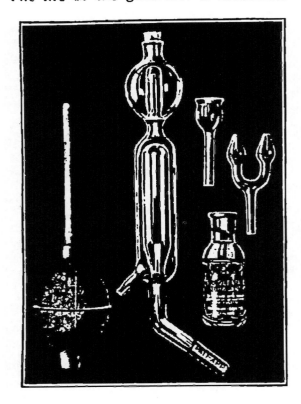

Instructions For Use Are Simple

The operation of High Frequency Violet Ray is simple, convenient, harmless to every age and condition, and painless. Where a counterirritant effect is required there is a stimulating sensation, but no pain. While every adult member of the family should serve their own needs, intelligent application of treatment and care of instrument should be observed.

1. Attach to light socket, then turn on current by operation of knob control To right applies and increases current; left decreases and shuts off.

2. Unless otherwise directed, electrode No. 1 is always used. Insert and remove electrode in instrument with a slight turn to the right. Apply and remove electrode to and from body with quick motion. Thus applied and removed there is no "spark" or slight tingle felt with slow application.

3. Treatment may be through clothing or direct upon body. If through clothing regulate current to the thickness of clothing and to comfort of patient. Thick clothing or covering causes a longer "spark" and a counter irritant effect.

4. In giving the direct treatment, place metal electrode in hand, turn on current, and draw the current to any part of the body with the fingers. This method can be used for body massage, facial massage and scalp treatment. No. 1 electrode may be used instead of No. 6 although it is not so strong. Use lubricant for body treatments.

5. Orificial or internal electrodes must be lubricated. Vaseline is a good lubricant. These should always be inserted before current is applied and current cut off before removal. Keep them clean and sterile. With the usual care of glass articles boiling is safe, or Lysol may be used.

6. Do not operate instrument longer than fifteen minutes without twenty minute intermission for cooling; otherwise overheating coils may result in damage to instrument.

7. Do not use any tonic containing alcohol on the hair.

8. Start the treatment with a mild current and gradually increase.

9. When through using the machine be sure and turn off the current at the switch, or, better still, detach plug from socket. The current is not off when the adjusting screw is turned tight to the left. Although no current may be passing into the electrode, yet the current is passing through the coils and they will become overheated. Damage

Stimulates Circulation

resulting from this cause is only the result of carelessness and is not covered in our guarantee. The safest method is to unscrew the plug from the socket when the machine is not in use.

10. When inserting electrodes into the nozzle of the machine do not try to force them into the socket should they fit a little tight. Hold the electrode firmly in hand and while pushing it into the socket twist it a half turn to the right. This will help to spread the socket prongs and permit the electrode to slide in more readily. When removing the electrode twist it a trifle to the right as you pull on it. Nearly eighty percent of broken electrodes can be eliminated by following the above instructions carefully.

11. Electrodes other than those with instruments may be had as required. Those included in equipment serve the purpose of the average family use.

12. The suggestions for treatment on pages 3 to 10 are based upon clinical experience. The time required in each treatment is basically correct, but not inflexible. Also the terms, mild, medium and strong, relating to current are subject to judgment which a little experience will bring.

13. Remember that the primary purpose is to heat the tissues deeply. To effect this Electrode should be moved slowly over area treated and may be held stationary over most painful parts.

Consider These Reasons Why You Should Own a High Frequency Outfit

High Frequency treatments make you feel young, glowing with health, full of energy and enthusiasm. The effects are most invigorating and stimulating—and it's a joy you can provide at very small cost.

The everlasting usefulness is only one of the great advantages. The pages you have just read indicate how this High Frequency Generator can be beneficial to you—pain, run down condition and non-active unhealthful body cells just can't resist the searching rays of this helpful device.

. . . .and it's so easy to use—so harmless that it's safe for a child and an actual pleasure to use it.

The High Frequency Generator itself is of exclusive scientific design and the electrodes are a masterpiece of therapeutic craftsmanship.

Here indeed is the long looked for, low cost High Frequency Generator for the home. Compact, Substantial, Dependable. have one of your own and use it as directed and you'll find that improvement in health will result.

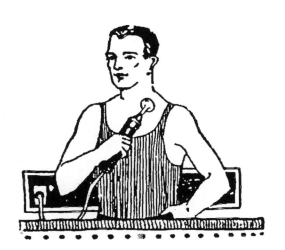

Produces   Muscular   And   Cellular   Massage

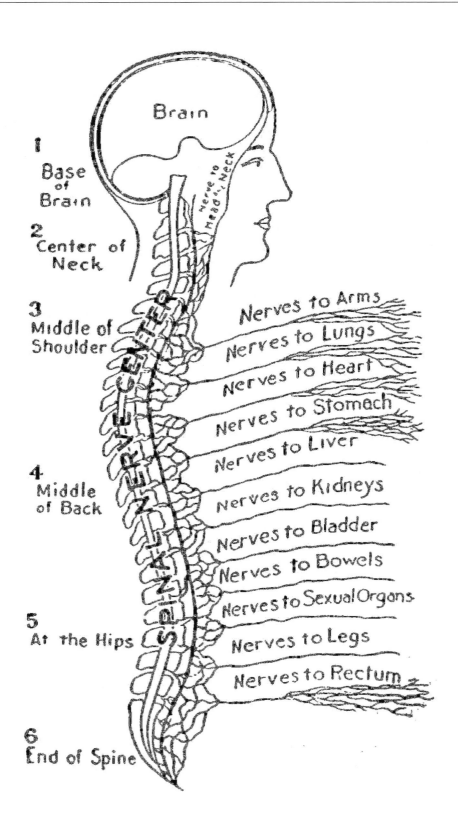

CHAPTER IV

Halliwell Shelton

High Frequency Violet Ray

For

Beauty and Better Health

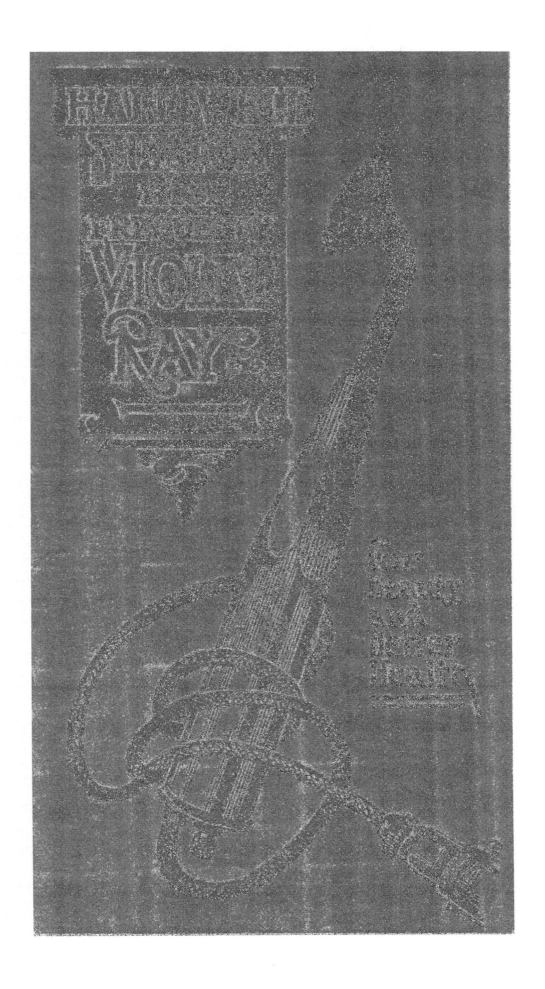

The
Halliwell Shelton Violet Ray
High Frequency Generator

Is the result of years of experience and experimentation on the part of expert engineers. The Halliwell Shelton Violet Ray Generator is as perfect as experience and workmanship can make it and is designed for both professional and home use. It is recommended, used and approved by the medical profession.

This Violet Ray Generator is the finest article of its kind manufactured in the world. Like the Shelton Vibrator, which is the acknowledged leader of the Vibrator field, the Halliwell Shelton Violet Ray Generator is the leader of the Violet Ray world.

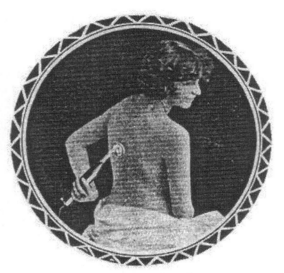

VITALITY - PHYSICAL DEVELOPMENT

The Violet Ray can be used by anyone, anywhere. Its construction is simple; its design is appealing, its workmanship is of the best, and the results it gives are vouched for by thousands, who have benefited by its use.

In brief, the Halliwell Shelton Violet Ray makes it possible for everyone to enjoy right at home the energizing, health-giving and pain-relieving powers of this wonderful ray.

GUARANTEE
All Halliwell Shelton Violet Ray Generators are guaranteed for a period of one year against electrical and mechanical imperfections.

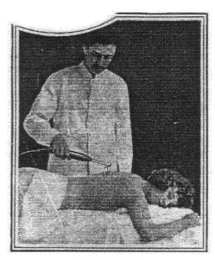

NEURITIS

Is an inflamed condition of the nerves. Any nerve can be affected. Pain and tenderness extend usually over the whole diseased nerve trunk. A mild current should be used at first and electrode kept in close contact with the body, moving it lightly. In some cases an increase of the pain may be noted at beginning. However, this state is soon overcome, then a more powerful spray can be applied.

Effects from Violet Ray treatments are systemic and not only local. Therefore all treatments have a fundamental action on health and benefit nerves and nerve endings.

What the Violet Ray Is

The Violet Ray High Frequency Current, or as it is more commonly called, the "Violet Ray," is a new phase of electricity. It is applied to any part of the human body without pain, muscular contraction or disagreeable sensation of any kind. The electrical oscillations representing the High Frequency Current follow each other with such tremendous rapidity that they outspeed our nervous sensibility; we do not become conscious of their presence; in other words: our nerves are insensitive to the electrical oscillations of the Violet Ray. The oscillations are so rapid that they exceed many hundred thousand repetitions per second. The Violet Rays are pleasing, and though most stimulating and highly invigorating to the entire system, nerves or muscles, cannot record the presence of their great power.

What Violet Rays Do

Violet Rays or High Frequency Currents benefit all living matter. Through the glass vacuum applicator light, heat, electric energy and ozone are created. These forces are uniformly potent in relieving and eliminating human ailments. Violet Rays present a remedy upon which we can rely. They are positive and certain in action. They will reach where medicine does not, and often cannot – yet they cause no pain, no disagreeable sensation or discomfort. They furnish a soothing relief. They destroy germs and have a strong power over infection.

A Violet Ray treatment is the surest method of relieving pain. Applied to that part of the body where the pain is severest, the rays and High Frequency electrical discharge penetrate every cell, tissue and organ and tranquilize and soothe. They build up the forces of nutrition and general health. Violet Rays will stimulate and strengthen the vital organs, develop the body and steady the nerves, spraying thousands of volts of High Frequency electricity into any weak, sluggish or painful organ or muscle, purifying and causing the flood of warm, rich blood to surge through the treated part, at the same time being painless and pleasant. Violet Rays have only to be tried to be appreciated.

Violet Rays for Well People, Too

Even if you are at present strong and well in every respect, the use of Violet Rays will be of immense benefit to you. They provide a stimulation to which a healthy body immediately responds. They safeguard you against the coming illness and reduction of vitality.

Why You Should Use Violet Rays

Violet Rays should be used by everyone experiencing sickness or ailments of any kind.

The healing properties of Violet Rays are manifold, and they accomplish what drugs and medicines never can. The regular introduction of a vitalizing shower of diffused electricity into your system is exactly what is needed to make it function properly and efficiently.

No matter how well you may be feeling today, tomorrow may bring sickness. But if you have been taking regular treatments with Violet Rays the chances that you will succumb to illness are very slight. Violet Ray treatments keep your constitution at "par."

The healthiest people in the world are those who are always striving to better their physical conditions. And there is nothing like a Violet Ray treatment to infuse vitality and energy into your body.

To be healthy, use Violet Rays. To keep healthy, use Violet Rays.

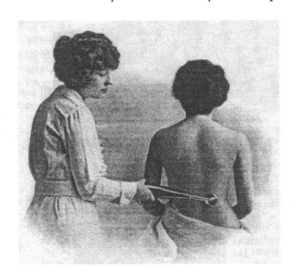

KIDNEY TROUBLES

The kidneys perform a very important task in our body. They are the organs of excretion. If their function is somehow impaired by inflammation due to heavy cold or due to congestion or other causes, grave con-sequences are resultant.

Violet Rays exert a powerful influence. The very fact that albumen in the urine quickly disappears after a few applications alone proves sufficiently their importance in fighting this class of sickness. Nobody who suffers from kidney disorders can really afford to be without a Violet Ray. It helps when other means, especially drugs, have long been given up as useless.

To Relieve Pains Use the Following Technique

Always apply as much of a current strength as can be tolerated. If a person is very sensitive, keep the electrode in close contact with the painful spot and move it slowly about. If the sufferer from pain does not object to it, treat through clothing or a towel and cause a counter irritation by sparks. It depends largely on the part or area you treat what method should be employed. It is therefore necessary to adapt yourself to circumstances.

Many people, after stopping their treatments for many weeks, and even months, report continual increase in health and strength. As a matter of fact, the greatest benefit comes after the course of treatment is over. This answers the question often asked as to whether the treatment does not have to be kept up indefinitely.

Orificial Treatments

All orificial electrodes must be lubricated before insertion. They should be properly sterilized. It is wrong to believe that orificial treatments are painful. There is, in fact, no other sensation than that of a beneficial warmth during the application. Orificial treatments do not last over 5 minutes. It is also advisable to move the electrode during the treatment just slightly so as to avoid its sticking to the mucous membrane. Orificial treatments require, for safety's sake and for better results, always two people, patient and operator. Always turn the current on after insertion of the applicator and turn the current off before removing the same.

Preparation for Treatment

Surface treatments can be given in direct contact with the skin, and also through the clothing. As any clothing represents an interposed dry resistance, a treatment through the same would cause small sparks. It depends entirely on the desired effect, which way to treat, and the instructions given in our booklet refer to the proper technique. If no sparks are desired any clothing covering the part to be treated must be removed.

Metallic objects as hairpins, corset steels, chains, should be taken off if they cannot be avoided in the treatment.

For Mild Treatments

Keep the applicator in close contact with the body at any part which requires a mild treatment.

Start with the weakest current possible. Avoid the initial little discharge which occurs when you bring the applicator close to the body in making the contact. Make contact quickly and the initial discharge will not be annoying. Do the same when the treatment is finished. Remove the electrode quickly. This will save you the little sparks you may otherwise feel. By no means does this little spark, when making contact with the applicator and when removing it, hurt. If you think it does, it is imaginary. Just use common sense and a little judgment and you will find that even one-half inch of High Frequency discharge does not cause any pain.

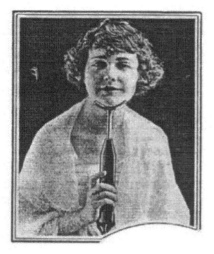

GOITRE

By using the No. 5 Electrode, throat and neck may be treated with admirable results. Many physicians recommend this treatment for Goitre.

Many cases yield to treatment using Electrode No. 5 with the strongest current that can be tolerated. Treatments should be of not longer than four minutes' duration and not more than once a day. Results are not usually apparent until a dozen or more treatments have been taken.

For sore throats, also for improvement of the voice, the surface applicator can be used. Singers, actors and speakers have reported wonderful improvement and benefits.

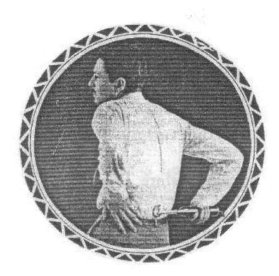

BACKACHE

Backache, except in cases of strain or internal injury, is a symptom of some internal disorder such as lumbago and rheumatism or weak sexual organs, bladder or kidneys. Local applications will relieve immediate pain but the cause should be located and treatment applied. Relief from the above ailments is usually obtained most quickly by local application on the affected area, using the Surface Electrode with fairly strong current.

For tired, wornout, rundown feeling, often accompanied by headache, nothing is more appropriate and relieving than Violet Ray treatments. They re-vitalize the system and reestablisb the correct vital functions of the body.

Ozone Generator

This instrument when attached to our Generator produces enormous quantities of Ozone which is purified by passing through the inhalant mixture provided with this attachment. A few drops of the inhalant are poured on the cotton, and when the rubber bulb is agitated, the Ozone is forced through this mixture and inhaled in the form of a vapor.

When using the Ozone Generator, support the instrument on a table so that it will not roll and insert the Ozone Generator the same as any other electrode. One hand must be in contact with the glass stem of the Ozone Generator as in the illustration.

The Ozone permeates every cell in the lungs, destroying any germ life and soothing the inflamed tissues. For Anemia, Hay Fever, Coughs, Catarrh, Asthma, Bronchitis, Insomnia, Nervous Debility and Tuberculosis of the Lungs, there is no better treatment.

The treatments are exceedingly agreeable and remind one of a trip to the pine woods.

No. 28 Ozone Generator. Price, complete with all the attachments and 1-ounce bottle of inhalant. **$10.00**

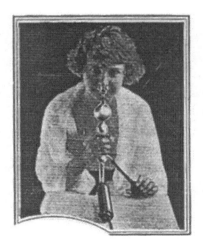

What the Ozone Treatment Will Do For You

If you lack physical exercise a good number of so-called functional troubles (of men and women of the sedentary class) will gradually make their appear-

OZONE GENERATOR

This style Ozone electrode can be attached to all Halliwell Shelton Violet Ray Outfits excepting Nos. 205 and 206, which contain built-in attachments.

Treatment not over 5 to 10 inhala-tions at one time. Use twice a day.

The Violet Ray Book

ance. These are clearly due to under-oxygenation, which means that an insufficient quantity of oxygen is absorbed by our system.

Muscular exercise, deep breathing, will increase oxygenation and do wonders to us, – as is well known – but how often can the person' needy of plenty of exercise, have same, especially when professional occupation and duties offer little chance for it? There are also a good many who may be invalid and should not exert themselves by physical strain. For all of these the Ozone Treatments will do wonders.

The Ozone Generator converts the oxygen of the air into ozone. Ozone, therefore, is a modification of oxygen; in fact, it is concentrated oxygen. It has a strong chemical action. It is a colorless gas which has a peculiar, not unpleasant, odor.

Ozone exists in larger quantities on mountain tops, at the Sea Shore and in the Country. In cities, and especially in crowded places, it is hardly recognizable. Oxygen is – as we all know – most vital to our welfare; in fact, without it we could not exist. When life is at its lowest ebb in grave cases of sickness the physicians resort to the oxygen tank to keep us breathing and alive. It is therefore not difficult to realize of what great importance ozone, which is concentrated oxygen, can be to us.

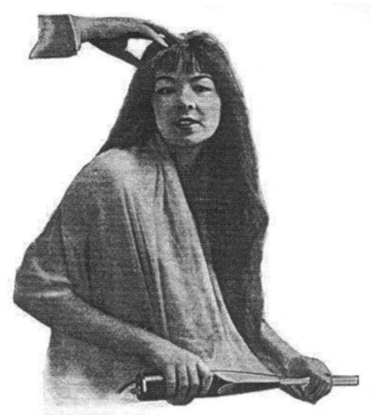

Indirect Massage

High Frequency current produces a cellular massage, the contractile effect being expended upon the individual cells composing the tissue rather than on the individual muscles. This form of massage is very effective, penetrating as it does every part of the body, and can be drawn to any desired part by the application of another person's fingers to the part of the body to which treatment is particularly desired, the patient first grasping the electrode as shown in above illustration.

No. 6 Electrode is especially designed for this treatment.

You can, however, use No. 1 with very good results; current not so strong, however. Where a very powerful treatment is wanted the metal Electrode No. 6 is used, but to avoid the sting turn the current on and off while the person treated has hand on the metal Electrode as illustrated.

Effects Desired Easily Obtained

Careful study of different ways of administration should be made before using Violet Ray so as to secure best results.

For sedative or quieting results, your entire body can be thoroughly charged with Violet Ray High Frequency current. You can completely electrify yourself. Painful sensations by sedative treatments can be calmed, as sedative action is strongly constitutional in its effects. Nervous ailments are greatly benefited by sedative treatments. They tranquilize your nerves. By keeping the electrode in close contact with part to be treated sedation can be produced locally. Sedative current creates quick and beneficial results in all nervous conditions. The entire nervous System is refreshed with a general electrification treatment.

Violet Ray can be stimulative. When an electrode is somewhat lifted during the application or used through clothing or cloth, a general stimulation is produced. This stimulation is caused by the many small sparks generally called High Frequency Spray. They cause a pleasant and tingling sensation and bombard thoroughly the area which they cover, causing a very beneficial heating effect at the same time. They also generate ozone which is directly driven into the tissue, causing the ozonization of the blood. These sparks are also germ-killing and overcome infection.

Follow Instructions Carefully

It is necessary to give strict attention to the following instructions to receive benefits – if same are followed, excellent results will positively be obtained.

ABSCESSES – Keep electrode No. 1 in close contact with the skin. Use enough current to get the full effect of the heat generated. Treatment of 3 to 5 minutes' duration and repeat daily or twice a day, if necessary. If applied to a developing abscess, its growth can be arrested.

ACNE (PIMPLES, BLACKHEADS) – A common and very distressing condition in young people, one in which quick and permanent relief may be obtained by the use of a short spark. Treat the entire surface for about six minutes, using electrode No. 1. Use electrode No. 46, creating a mild fulguration spark where blackheads are deeply imbedded in the tissues, thus softening and permitting their easy removal. Steaming the face before treatment will be found beneficial. During period of treatments diet should be carefully regulated, avoid rich and greasy foods, and keep bowels in a healthy condition.

ALOPECIA (LOSS OF HAIR) – Commence treatment with weak current and increase to medium strength later, by using electrode No. 3. Pass comb electrode back and forth over scalp for about four minutes every day. Use same treatment for baldness due to sickness and for gray hair in order to restore it to natural condition. Electrodes No. 1 or No. 5 can be used if more convenient.

ALCOHOLISM AND DRUG ADDICTIONS – Use surface electrode No. 1 in alcohol, morphine or opium habits, apply a strong current over liver, solar plexus and spine, for six to eight minutes daily. In cocaine habits use a mild current to the soles of the feet, arms and legs until reddening results. These applications should be made through interposed towel or clothing. Short sparks are best for these treatments. Never apply current through shoes.

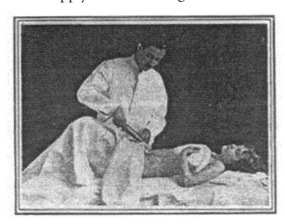

ANEMIA

Surface Electrode should he applied to the naked body over the chest, abdomen, back, and particularly up and down the entire spine. This will have a general stimulating effect through the increase of the oxygenation of the blood. In this way the oxygen-carrying powers of the red blood corpuscles are increased.

ANEMIA AND CHLOROSIS – Use electrode No. 1 for eight to ten minutes three to six times per week, treating thoroughly the entire chest, abdomen, back and spine, thus increasing the oxygenation of the blood, which is as effective as iron tonics to the system. Ozone inhalations are helpful and of utmost value in these cases. Use Ozone Generator No. 28.

ARTERIOSCLEROSIS AND HIGH BLOOD PRESSURE – Daily treatments of about 8 minutes' duration will lower blood pressure. As the blood approaches normal, reduce treatments to three a week, then to twice a week. A treatment every week or two should be maintained for some time to be sure of the permanency of results. Apply electrode No. 1 or No. 2, using a medium current strength over the body generally.

ASTHMA – In asthmatic conditions, the best results may be obtained through the use of the Ozone Generator, electrode No. 28. Choking and coughing fits will be promptly alleviated. A local auxiliary treatment may also be used for a sedative effect by a gentle massage over the area with the surface electrode No. 1 and mild current. Also apply electrode No. 5 to throat glands for about 6 minutes.

ATAXIA – Use a sharp spark along the spine, over buttocks, abdomen and to the back of the legs. Apply electrode No. 1 or No. 4. Daily treatments lasting about 10 minutes are necessary at first. They can be gradually decreased to about two a week with the progressing improvements.

BACKACHE – To relieve pain treat sore muscles with electrode No. 1. As backache may be due to weakness of the bladder or sexual organs, lumbago, rheumatism, kidney disease, it is important to treat the cause as well.

BARBER'S ITCH (CYCOSIS) – Cleanse the infected area with warm water and castile soap, and a mild antiseptic wash. Then treat with mild current from the surface electrode No. 1 in close contact, followed by a short spark till counter-irritation is produced. The condition is usually stubborn and may require extended treatment.

BLADDER DISEASE (CYSTITIS) – The result of vacuum tube treatment through the rectum or urethral is remarkable in inflammation of the bladder. Treatment lasting 7 minutes given daily at first and then every other day, will clear up urine very fast in nearly all of these cases. Use electrodes No. 1 or No. 2.

BRONCHITIS – Short sparks applied with electrode No. 1 or No. 2 over the chest and back, until well reddened, will give relief. This treatment may be repeated every hour until a sufficient moderation of congestion is obtained. More important than the high frequency application is to ozonize the air by means of electrode No. 28.

BRAIN FAG – Use electrode No. 1 over the forehead and eyes and to the back of the head and neck with spark just strong enough to have good tonic effect. In all cases, 2 or 3 minutes' inhalation of ozone (electrode No. 28) is desirable.

BREAST DEVELOPMENT – Treat the entire area to be developed. Use electrode No. 1 for about 5 to 8 minutes daily. Move it lightly over each side, from the neck downward and also from arm pit to arm pit, under each breast, pressing lightly upward.

BRIGHT'S DISEASE – Apply strong current with electrode No. 1 over the region of the kidneys for at least 10 minutes every day.

BRUISES – Treat injured area with electrode No. 1. First with close contact and later with gradually increasing spark. Use lubricant.

BUNIONS – Electrode No. 18 or No. 51, using a fairly strong current, should be applied directly over the inflamed area followed by a gentle spark.

CALLOUSES – On calloused areas of foot a mild fulguration spark obtained from electrode No. 20 will soften the hardened tissues so they can be readily removed. If soreness follows, treatment over the area with the surface electrode No. 1 in direct contact with the skin will afford relief.

CANCER – Mild forms of cancer are treated with a strong spark. Use electrode No. 20. Consult authority, as surgery is usually required in conjunction.

CANKER – A medium current for 1 or 2 minutes should be applied with electrode No. 10 or No. 58, or any suitable dental electrode.

CARBUNCLES – Use electrode No. 1 in loose contact with the inflamed area and pass it back and forth over it for 5 to 10 minute. This will relieve pain and promote an early ripening of the carbuncle. Electrode No. 18 is also very convenient.

CATARRHAL CONDITIONS – In catarrh of the nose and throat the ozone generator No. 28 is of great value and should be used two or three times daily for about 5 minutes at a time, followed by treatment in the nostrils with the nasal electrode No. 16 or 52 with mild current for about 3 minutes. Care should be used that the current is not turned on until after insertion of the electrode.

CATARACT – Five minutes daily treatments with electrode No. 18 in contact with closed eyelids, with not too great an intensity of current.

CHAFE – Use vaseline, followed by a medium current with electrode No. 1 for 5 to 6 minutes in close contact with skin.

CHAPPED HANDS OR FACE – Apply vaseline first. Then use a weak current with No. 1 electrode for 2 minutes in contact with skin.

CHILBLAINS – Use electrode No. 1 for 6 to 8 minutes in contact with the skin. It may he held steadily over the chilblain or moved slowly about as desired. Repeat daily or every other day until cured.

COLD HANDS OR FEET – Improper circulation in the extremities may be relieved by a gentle spark over their surface, gradually increasing until a sense of warmth prevails. Use electrode No. 2. Repeat often; if necessary, three times a day.

COLDS – Cold in the head will be benefited by inhalation from ozone generator (electrode No. 28), followed by mild current through nasal electrode No. 52. The surface electrode No. 1 may also be used over the antrum, mastoid region, and back of neck.

COLD IN LUNGS – Treat the chest and back. Follow instructions given under Asthma. Take ozone inhalations repeatedly for several minutes. Electrode No. 28.

CONSTIPATION – Relief will be obtained by a thorough downward massage over the abdominal region with surface electrode No. 1 applied first directly to the skin and followed by short spark over the same area. Ten minutes daily is advised first, later dropping to two or three times a week. If the constipation is particularly stubborn, peristaltic action will be stimulated by means of the insertion of an insulated rectal electrode (Nos. 14, 34, 36 or 63), properly lubricated, for a period of 4 to 6 minutes. Apply current after insertion.

CORNS – Hard corns may be entirely removed by the application of the fulguration electrodes Nos. 18 or 51, care being used to apply the spark particularly upon the hard tissue and not on the surrounding area.

DANDRUFF – Shampoo the scalp before treatment, dry it thoroughly and apply a medium current, with applicator No. 3, using it in the same manner as an ordinary comb for 3 to 5 minutes. Repeat this treatment at intervals of 2 to 3 days. Do not use any hair tonic.

DEAFNESS – Unless the drum of the ear is ruptured, chronic deafness may generally be relieved and in many cases entirely cured by high frequency treatment. Ear electrode No. 10 should be used for about 4 minutes. The gentle stimulation thus afforded the delicate aural nerves and the mild massage of the drum will often result in an immediate improvement in hearing. As a further treatment the surface electrode may be applied over the mastoid region for 2 or 3 minutes with a gentle, mild current.

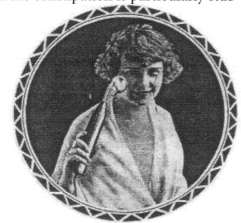

FOR THE COMPLEXION

There is no more delightful or effective method of removing blemishes or wrinkles and other complexion disorders than by Violet Ray treatment. The blood is brought to the surface and the bloom of youth and health is restored to the cheeks. Skin-troubles, Acne, Pimples and Eczema respond quickly to Violet Rays. No beauty specialist is nowadays without a Violet Ray outfit.

DIABETES – Apply, electrodes Nos. 1 and 2 over the abdomen, and if proper diet is observed, results will be quickly obtained. Apply a strong current for about 8 minutes through a thin towel twice a day.

DIPHTHERIA – Apply electrodes Nos. 10 and 58 to inside and outside of throat respectively. Ozone inhalations have proven most beneficial (Ozone Generator No. 28).

DYSPEPSIA – Apply surface electrode No. 1 over stomach and solar plexus. The great tonic effect of ozone inhalations makes it a useful adjunct.

EARACHE – Relief obtained by application of ear electrode No. 10, using a mild current for 3 to 5 minutes. Applications to the back of the ear and over the side of the face covering facial nerve with electrode No. 1 assist treatment greatly.

ECZEMA – A handkerchief laid over the surface will cause a slight spark and is preferable. If the skin itches hold the electrode slightly away from the surface. This will relieve and gratify. Use electrode No. 1 or No. 18.

EYE DISEASES – Iritis, retinitis, atrophy of optic nerve, conjunctivitis, trachoma, glaucoma, incipient cataract, paralysis of ocular muscles, intro-ocular hemorrhage have all been treated by high frequency currents. Close eyelids and apply a mild current with electrode No. 18 or No. 39 for short periods, not exceeding 3 minutes at one time.

FELONS – Treat with No. 1 electrode and a mild current in close contact daily from 4 to 6 minutes.

FEMALE TROUBLES – Use electrodes Nos. 13, 30 or 31. They should be lubricated before insertion. Turn the current on after insertion of electrode and turn the current off before removing to avoid unnecessary sparking. A medium current for 5 minutes is applied. Repeat treatment as circumstances require. During menstruation an excessive flow of blood may result, as high frequency currents draw the blood.

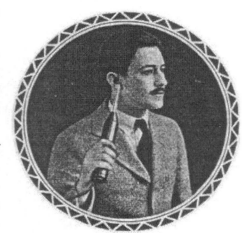

FOR THE EAR

Is an inflamed condition of the nerves. Any nerve can be affected. Pain and Earache, deafness and other disorders of the auditory organs yield readily to the Violet Ray. In some cases, hearing has been restored completely.

Use Electrode No. 10, inserting it into the ear, using a mild current for a short length of time. Where the pain is acute it is sometimes necessary to take hourly applications. If heating effect is too marked during treatment interrupt the application and repeat later.

When inflammation exists treat about the ear with No. 1 Electrode from 5 to 6 minutes with mild current.

FISTULAS – Use electrode Nos. 14, 36 or 63, as indicated. Lubricate electrode before insertion into rectum. Use a medium current for about 5 minutes daily.

FLABBY BREAST – A stimulating application with the surface electrode to the relaxed nipple of the flabby breast will immediately show its beneficial effect.

FRECKLES – Several weeks' treatment will be required. Use electrode No. 1 with a medium current daily from 4 to 6 minutes.

FROST BITES – Treat affected part with No. 1 electrode, using a mild current for from 5 to 7 minutes.

FURUNCULOSIS – Treat with No. 1 electrode with mild or medium current. Inflammation will cease quickly.

GOITRE – The absorption of tissue being necessary, treat with external throat electrode No. 5 in close contact with the skin and follow with moderately sharp spark over the surface and sides of the protuberance. Persistence in this treatment is necessary.

GOUT – This condition may be helped by a continued massage over the area with a surface electrode and a mild current. If pain is felt at first begin with short treatment and increase. Do not treat during acute attack.

GRAY HAIR – The natural color of hair can often be restored by patient treatments with electrode No. 3. See under Alopecia. Sometimes several months are required for results. Keep the scalp clean. Use a current of sufficient strength for good stimulation once or twice every day.

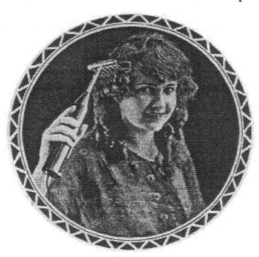

SCALP TREATMENT

Nothing is more beneficial to the scalp than the application of the Violet Ray. It revitalizes impoverished hair, restores its natural lustre. In order to obtain results it is necessary to be both persistent and consistent in the use of Violet Ray, as treatments must sometimes continue over a long period of time in obstinate cases. Treatments should be from 3 to 5 minutes a day using the comb Electrode. Do not use hair tonic that contains alcohol, as this is inflammable. Falling hair can be stopped in time by Violet Ray scalp applications. Prematurely gray hair can be restored to its natural color by persistent applications. Dandruff and other scalp troubles are usually quickly relieved.

GRIPPE (INFLUENZA) – Treat spine, solar plexus, over eyes and sides of nose. Inhalations from Ozone Generator (No. 28) will greatly aid. Intra-nasal applications by electrode No. 52 are also beneficial.

HAY FEVER – Apply electrode No. 1 over the nose and the spine and No. 28 in nostrils. Anticipate the trouble and begin before discomfort is felt.

HEADACHES – Headaches are from varying causes. If relief is not had from applying to the seat of pain, cover the spine and stomach. Apply No. 1 electrode.

HIVES AND RASH – Use electrode No. 1 with medium current strength to affected area. Use vaseline before applying the electrode; 3 to 5 minutes should be sufficient. Repeat daily.

HEMORRHOIDS (PILES) – Use hemorrhoidal electrode No. 63 with mild current for about 4 to 6 minutes, care being observed that the electrode is properly lubricated and that current is not turned on until after insertion.

INSOMNIA – Cover back of head, neck and eyebrows in order mentioned. Use electrode No. 1; a strong current is essential in treating this ailment.

LEUCORRHEA – Follow the directions given under female troubles. Also use electrode No. 4, moving it up and down the spine slowly. A strong current must be used for about 5 to 6 minutes daily.

LUMBAGO – Treat over painful area until all pain is dispelled. Use electrode No. 1 and as strong a current as can be tolerated. Repeat treatment whenever pain reappears until cured.

MASSAGE – Metal electrode No. 6 to be held by patient in one hand, turning on current after it has been grasped. Masseur's fingers will draw sparks to point massaged. Use lubricant while massaging.

MUMPS – Treat the swollen parts with a medium current, using electrode No. 1, keeping it in contact for about 5 to 8 minutes. Repeat as necessary, at least once a day,

NERVOUSNESS – Treat the spine, back of head and neck with a mild current, using electrodes Nos. 1 and 4. Immediate results are felt in all cases. Use a weak current at first and increase the strength gradually; 5 to 8 minutes is the average duration of treatment.

NEURALGIA – Apply to seat of pain, after applying lubricant, raising electrode occasionally to produce spark. Treat with No. 1 electrode; time of treatment 5 to 10 minutes.

NEURITIS – The first few treatments usually increase the pain, after which relief is felt, and the current may be increased and a short spark given. Apply at the seat of pain with surface electrode No. 1.

OBESITY – Use electrode No. 1 and apply to affected parts consistently. Begin with a medium current and increase to full power. Rigorous diet, exercise and personal hygiene must, of course, be observed.

PAINS – Apply at seat of pain until relieved with current and method to give best results. Use electrode No. 1.

PARALYSIS – With electrodes No. 1 or No. 2 treat paralyzed muscles, employing a current strong enough to produce a half or three-quarter inch spark. Part of the time keep the applicator in contact with the skin and part of the time raise it above the surface to get effective spark.

POISON IVY – Apply lubricant first. Use No. 1 electrode or No. 2 edgewise so as to cause plenty of sparking over the whole affected area. Lift the applicator here and there and treat with a strong current for from 3 to 5 minutes.

PROSTATIC DISEASES – This most distressing ailment, common to so many men of middle age, is one in which the high frequency current is almost a specific. The treatment indicated is with the prostatic electrode No. 9. See Pages 14 and 15.

PYORRHEA – Treatments with suitable dental electrode with a weak or medium current will help to re-establish a healthy condition of the gums. High frequency treatments promote proper nutritional improvements and in addition to this have antiseptic and antitoxic properties. A dentist should always be consulted.

RED NOSE – Use electrode No. 1 and apply for short periods, say about 2 minutes, small sparks by holding the electrode edgeways or lifting it about one-eighth of an inch. The object is to destroy the enlarged veins and treatment must not be carried too far at one time. It should be repeated as condition permits. Several days between treatments may sometimes be advisable.

RHEUMATISM – High frequency currents are of exceptional value in muscular and in chronic articular rheumatism. The pain will be relieved by application of surface electrode No. 1 with massage, using lubricant, if necessary. Follow with fairly strong spark until pronounced redness is produced. This treatment persistently followed has in many cases resulted in a permanent cure. While relief may be obtained in one treatment, a permanent cure may require much time and patience.

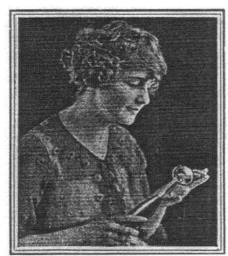

RHEUMATISM

There is no surer antidote on earth for rheumatism than Violet Ray treatment. In some cases rheumatism disappears almost completely after a few treatments.

RINGWORM – Use electrode No. 1 and apply short sparks for several minutes two or three times every other day. A medium current is sufficient. Move the electrode so as to cover the entire affected area.

SCARS – If the tissue is hardened or callous its removal may be facilitated by the application of a mild spark through electrode No. 20.

SCIATICA – Treat with a sharp spark along the course of the sciatic nerve until a redness is produced. Use electrode No. 1 or No. 2.

SKIN DISEASES – Treat over the affected tissues with surface electrode No. 1 held in close contact for from 5 to 15 minutes. Follow by moderate spark 3 to 5 minutes. Treat once daily. If the skin is moist, talcum powder should be used so that electrode will not stick. See also Acne and Eczema.

SORE FEET AND STONE BRUISES – Applications with any suitable applicator in close contact with the skin bring quick relief. Use lubricant and treat for several minutes.

SORE THROAT (TONSILITIS) – Electrode No. 5 is best suited for external throat applications. Hold directly against the skin with fairly strong current. The use of the Ozone Generator No. 28 for several minutes following will also be beneficial.

SPRAINS – The pain and soreness following a sprain may be alleviated by treatment, first with the surface electrode in contact with the skin and later by a mild spark, gradually increasing in strength until a hyperemia is produced.

STIFFNESS OF JOINTS AND MUSCLES – This condition is generally due to the over-employment of certain muscles. The resulting stiffness and soreness may be relieved by the use of surface electrode No. 1.

ULCERS – Apply a strong current with No. 2 electrode for 5 minutes in contact,

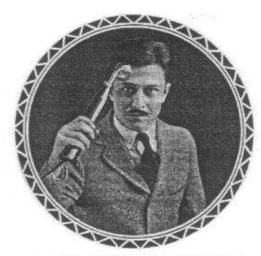

HEADACHE TREATMENT

lifting applicator once in a while to produce sparks of at least one-quarter inch. Repeat daily.

WARTS AND MOLES – These disfigurements, no matter of how long standing, may be most successfully treated by the application of a spark through the fulguration electrode No. 20. The greatest care must be exercised that these sparks do not come in contact with the surrounding tissues. Permanent results may be expected, and the most disfiguring warts or moles removed without leaving a trace by these means.

WHOOPING COUGH – Apply No. 1 electrode in the same manner as explained under Asthma and use also Ozone Inhalations with the Ozone Generator No. 28.

WRITER'S CRAMP – Treat with gentle spark over the affected fingers and thumb, also massage with surface electrode over palm of the hand.

WRINKLES – Are commonly caused by using a given set of facial muscles more than normally. They can be removed by applying electrode No. 1 or No. 18 with a rotary, massaging movement. With frequency current revitalizes tired muscles and arrests the blighting marks of time.

Medical authorities agree that 65% of all men past middle age (many much younger) are afflicted with a disorder of the prostate gland. Aches in feet, legs and back, sciatic pains, are some of the signs. No longer should a man approaching or past the prime of life be content to regard these pains and conditions as inevitable signs of approaching age. The Halliwell Shelton Violet Ray is used to restore youthful health and vigor and to restore the prostate gland to its proper functioning.

In treating the Prostate through the rectum the technique consists in placing the patient on one side in the Sims' position with the knees well drawn up. The No. 9 Electrode is lubricated, inserted in handle and then inserted into the rectum about six inches with the depression in the tube turned toward the front or anterior wall of the rectum so the gland rests into depression for best results. In Prostatic diseases of all kinds the High Frequency current has proven most efficacious. If, however, you are fortunate to have a Low frequency circuit in your machine, that is preferable in this treatment. For home use a two-piece machine is more desirable on account of the convenience of turning the current on and off. The duration of each treatment is 3 to 5 minutes. Results found in all forms of Prostate diseases are extraordinary. Enlarged Prostate should show improvement from the very first-about two to three treatments a week.

Same treatment used with remarkable results in Senile hypertrophy. Two or three treatments a week then skip a month.

Directions for Operation

1 – Insert the Glass Applicator into the handle of machine.

2 – Attach the plug to the lamp socket.

3 – Turn the current on: first, electric light switch; second, knob switch on machine.

4 – Turn the adjusting knob switch to the right or left also to increase or to diminish the Violet Ray discharge. Also give extra turn when finished to insure electric current is broken.

5 – In the indirect treatment, the party to be treated should hold the instrument, with the metal Electrode No. 6 attached in hand. The current should then be turned on and some second party, with either hand, fingertips or another applicator, draw the current to the desired spot of the patient's body. This method can be used for body Massage, facial massage and scalp treatment. No. 1 Applicator may be used in place of No. 6, although it is not so strong and desired results not so easily obtained.

6 – Do not attempt to repair instrument, if the necessity arises, but write to the factory, advising of your difficulties and we will inform you what to do.

7 – Do not use our instrument in connection with any tonic containing alcohol on the hair.

8 – Any treatment should be started with a mild current and gradually increased to the required strength.

9 – When a treatment is completed, do not forget to turn off the current at the switch, or to be on the safe side, remove plug from the electric light socket. Damage arising from carelessness is not covered in our guarantee.

10 – The standard winding for this instrument is 110 Volts. If voltage is higher or lower than 15 per cent, special windings or series resistances must be used to obtain the best results. We will supply all necessary information upon request.

11 – Take care of the connecting cords. They should be kept dry and free from knots and twists and must be repaired when signs of wear are apparent.

12 – Should you break the glass Electrode off in the machine accidentally, simply take a pair of long-nose plyers and pull out the broken part.

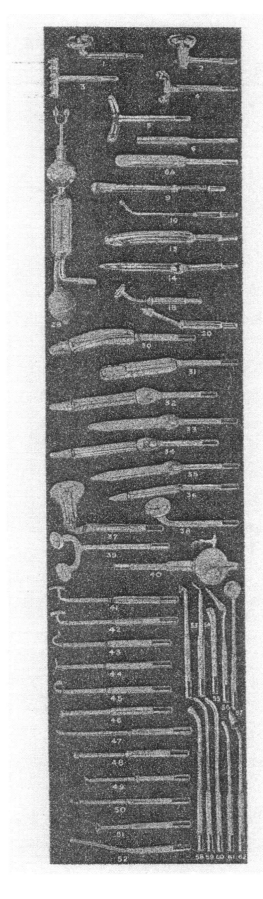

General High Frequency Electrodes

Made from the best annealed imported glass. Do not confuse the Halliwell-Shelton Electrodes with Electrodes made from plain glass

VIOLET RAY

No. 1—General surface for head, face or body $1.00
No. 2—Large condenser electrode, delivers strong current. For rheumatism, lumbago, etc. $3.00
No. 3—Large comb, scalp or body....$1.50
No. 3A—Derma Art Comb $1.50
No. 4—Spinal electrode $1.50
No. 5—External throat, arms, limbs $1.00
No. 6—Metal handle used for giving indirect treatment $1.25
No. 9—Insulated prostatic electrode..$2.00
No. 10—Ear or internal throat........$1.00
No. 13—Plain vaginal $1.00
No. 14—Plain rectal, small diameter..$1.00
No. 18—Eye electrode, also for corns.$1.00
No. 20—Fulguration electrode (or removal of warts, moles, diseased growths, etc. $2.00
No. 28—Ozone generator, with 1 oz. bottle of inhalant, nose and mouthpiece, and bulb $10.00
No. 30—Insulated vaginal electrode, large diameter $2.00
No. 31—Insulated vaginal electrode, generates ozone in vagina $3.00
No. 32—Insulated rectal, large diam..$2.00
No. 33—Plain rectal, large diam......$1.00
No. 34—Insulated rectal, med. diam..$2.00
No. 35—Plain rectal, medium diam...$1.00
No. 36—Insulated rectal, small $2.00
No. 37—Large kataphoric (cocaine) electrode—Medicated cotton inserted and high frequency applied through medicated contents. Particles of medicament are driven into tissue by molecular bombardment. Effect is purely local $4.00
No. 38—Hollow surface shaped, generates ozone within cavity and fits nicely over certain parts as cheek bones $1.25
No. 39—Double eye electrode $1.50
No. 40—Actinic ray electrode for acne vulgaris, ringworm, lupus, etc. Develops sufficient X-ray to cause actinic or chemical ray effect..................$10.00
No. 41—Dental electrode for gum treatment, right side of jaw........$2.00
No. 42—Dental electrode for gum treatment, left side of jaw........$2.00
No. 43—Dental electrode for gum treatment, inside of jaw................$2.00
No. 44—Dental electrode for front gum treatment $2.00
No. 45—Dental electrode, inside jaw..$2.00
No. 46—Insulated electrode, covers small area for pimples $2.00
No. 47—Dental kataphoric (cocaine) electrode $2.00
No. 48—Dental electrode for gum....$2.00
No. 49—Dental abscess electrode......$2.00
No. 50—Dental electrode ball shaped..$2.00
No. 51—Corn electrode $2.00
No. 52—Plain nasal electrode $1.00
No. 53—Dental electrode, hollow bulb $1.75
No. 54—Eyelid electrode $2.00
No. 55—Small kataphoric (cocaine) electrode. See No. 57..................$2.00
No. 56—Insulated ear electrode........$2.00
No. 57—Insulated spatulum or tongue $2.00
No. 58—Insulated internal throat $2.00
No. 59—Insulated urethral electrode $2.00
No. 60—Plain urethral $1.00
No. 61—Insulated nasal electrode......$2.00
No. 62—Dental fulguration electrode..$1.75
No. 63—Hemorrhoidal $1.00

NEON ELECTRODE PRICES

All regular Violet Ray Electrodes as listed above at $1.00 each can be supplied in Neon at $3.00 each.

All regular Violet Ray Electrodes as listed above at $1.75 and $2.00 each can be supplied in Neon at $4.00 each.

CHAPTER V

RenuLife Electric Company

Violet Ray

For

Health, Strength, Beauty

Health

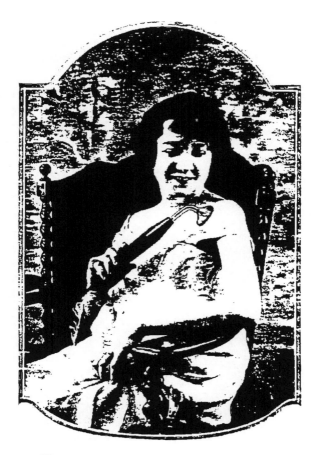

RenuLife

VIOLET RAY

Health – Strength – Beauty

High Frequency Violet Ray Simply Explained

High Frequency electric current has an entirely different effect on the human body than the crude, shocking sensation produced by ordinary electric current. There is no shock, pain or muscular contraction from the Violet Ray High Frequency current. The ordinary house lighting current is completely modified. Its volume or amperage is reduced to a low measure, while the pressure, or voltage is tremendously increased and the number of oscillations raised exceedingly high. When this modified current is applied to the human body, the nerves are insensible to the electric waves because of their enormous rapidity of movement. The Renulife High Frequency current is pleasant and painless, yet penetrative and effective.

High Frequency treatments are applied by a vacuum glass tube called an Electrode, in which the High Frequency current shows in a violet colored glow. From this phenomenon the common name Violet Ray is derived.

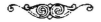

Increase Your Efficiency Through a Course of Renulife High Frequency Treatments

The stimulating effects of the Renulife Violet Ray are of inestimable benefit to the modern business or professional man who, cooped up in an office or store all day, has not the time for gymnastics or systematic physical exercise. Sitting in a chair for hours at a time, his circulation becomes sluggish, the poisons are not eliminated properly from the body and the nerve force is used more rapidly than it is renewed. A run-down, tired-out condition results, which lowers general working efficiency and takes the edge off mental alertness and physical vigor.

Page One

Renulife VIOLET RAY *for*

For that Tired. Worn-Out. Run-Down Feeling

Some constitutions will stand much more abuse than others. Persistent overwork will break down the strongest constitution. You notice a lessening of your animal spirits; you realize that there is a limit to your endurance; your appetite is not good; your back aches; you have dizzy spells when you stoop; you have pains in your chest and shoulders; your food does not digest; your bowels are irregular; and you do not get rest from your sleep but awaken tired; you are dull and without your old ambition; your vital force is low—in fact your reserve strength is gone, and your resistance is breaking down.

Nature will repair the damage if you give her the right aid.

Get your blood circulating properly again. Tone and restore the quality of the blood, tissues and nerves. With a Renulife you can stimulate and revitalize your entire system reestablish healthy circulation, and set all the vital functions in robust action.

How Renulife Benefits the Ailing

It is extremely doubtful whether any of the manifold uses of electricity has proven more beneficial to mankind than its application to the healing art.

The Violet Ray is a thorough treatment; the irresistible, revitalizing powers of the Violet Ray being carried at once to every nerve cell. fiber and part of the body; even the heart is saturated It increases the oxygen in the blood, enriching and purifying it, and giving added vitality and strength, and so eliminates the poisonous waste products to which much disease is due. It exercises without effort or the weakening waste of energy The Violet Ray reaches and treats the cause of the disease whether known or not, and so strikes at the very root of the disturbance.

The Renulife Violet Ray High Frequency current produces a cellular massage. Instead of the contraction of muscles, the individual cells are stimulated by the oscillation of the electric current. This causes a marked improvement in nutrition and general health. The benefits are not confined to the local area or part, but are constitutional in results.

Health – Strength – Beauty

Location of Vital Organs

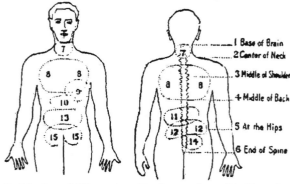

1 Base of Brain
2 Center of Neck
3 Middle of Shoulder
4 Middle of Back
5 At the Hips
6 End of Spine

7. Neck and Throat 10. Stomach 13. Bowels
8. Lungs   11. Liver   14. Spleen
9. Heart   12. Kidneys 15. Loins

Renulife Applied at These Vital Seats is a Most Effective Agent in Restoring Normal Functioning

Beneficial Effects of Renulife Violet Ray

1. Increased blood supply to a given area.
2. Increased oxygen in the blood.
3. Increased elimination of waste products.
4. Increased bodily heat without a corresponding rise in temperature.
5. Destruction of germs.
6. Mild sparks stimulate or soothe according to length and character of application.
7. Lower blood pressure.
8. Soothing of nerves.

Drives Out Pains and Aches

Aches and pains are messages from some troubled organ, muscle or nerve It is a call for relief. It may be the stomach is in distress with an overtaxing load, or the bowels congested, or the nervous system in general reacting against some abuse. The pain or ache may be localized. while the cause originated in a remote functional relation.

A pain in an arm is likely to be the local manifestation of a blood stream laden with poison, which has also affected the nerves and the result is Rheumatism.

The Violet Ray is the most potent pain and ache eradicator. because while it breaks up local congestions, stimulating circulation, at the same time it acts directly on the blood. A baptism of ozone purifies the blood relieving nerve pressure. Pains and aches vanish.

Renulife VIOLET RAY for

Some Uses of Renulife Violet Ray

In this booklet no attempt is made to give full directions for using Renulife Violet Ray. The treatment chart and directions for operating accompanying each instrument take up in detail just how to secure the best results in treating each of the ailments enumerated. Renulife Models and Electrodes are shown on pages 21 - 28. Diseases are discussed in alphabetical order. The testimonials are taken from unsolicited letters sent us by Renulife users.

ACNE (Pimples)

Renulife Violet Ray is a boon to those afflicted with Acne. The disfigurement of a pimply skin can be overcome by using Electrode No. 1 over the affected surface for from seven to ten minutes, three to six times a week.

"I am now entirely relieved of Acne, which I have been treating with your Violet Ray, and I see no symptoms of its return."

ALOPECIA (Falling Hair)

Falling hair is usually caused by improper circulation of the blood. Renulife Violet Ray scalp treatments insure proper nourishment of the scalp and consequently are beneficial in the treatment of dandruff, falling hair, gray hair and itching scalp.

"After using your Violet Ray Generator for a short time, I wish to tell you that it has completely cured me of falling hair and dandruff. I notice also that it is restoring my hair to its natural color."

ANEMIA (Lack of Red Corpuscles in Blood)

When the Renulife Violet Ray is applied to the body, two things result: Increased circulation of the blood and by actual count, an increased number of red blood corpuscles. The result is extremely beneficial in all cases of Anemia, Chlorosis and Arteriosclerosis (Hardening of the Arteries).

"I have a girl 12 years old, who has been sick for two years, and I find that she is getting more help from the Violet Ray than the best doctors can do for her. She is Anemic and has been unable to sleep. But after five months' treatment she sleeps all night without waking up. We are in hopes she can go to school again soon."

Health–Strength–Beauty

ASTHMA

Asthma is treated with Electrode No. 1 in light contact over the chest and throat glands, and over the shoulder blades down as far as the waist. Ozone inhalations supplement this treatment. Hundreds of Asthma sufferers have found relief with Violet Ray.

"My son had Chronic Bronchial Asthma. Every time we had rainy or foggy weather these attacks came on. He could scarcely breathe. Since taking Renulife Ozone treatments he has had but one slight attack. Since then he has not been troubled with Asthma and I find his breathing is so much better."

BLADDER DISEASE (Cystitis)
(Inflammation of the Bladder)

Vacuum tube treatment has been found to produce remarkable results in cases of inflammation of the bladder. Treatment may be given daily, or in acute cases every four hours. Results usually follow in short order. Treat locally over the bladder and lower spine with Electrode No. 1 using a strong current with light contact. In women, treat through the vagina with Electrode No. 9, thereby getting the current to the neck of the bladder. In men or in young girls, use Electrode No. 7 in the rectum.

"I have scored another success with my Model 'R' Renulife. Last Saturday I was taken with a hemorrhage of the bladder. My doctor suggested that I try No. 27 Electrode. I followed the directions and next morning there was no trace of trouble. I feel rather wonderful about it."

BOILS

Boils are successfully treated with medium to strong Renulife current for seven or eight minutes twice a day. Where a boil has started it can often be stopped by the Violet Ray current. If it cannot be stopped it will come to a head much quicker and the pain will be greatly relieved.

"A man came to me with a big boil on his forearm, and his arm was so lame he could not lift it. I gave him a treatment with my Violet Ray machine, and the next day the boil was gone, and the soreness was all gone out of his arm. This shows you what Violet Ray will do."

BRONCHITIS

Very beneficial results can be obtained with Violet Ray in the treatment of Bronchitis, especially when the Ozone attachment is also used.

RenuLife VIOLET RAY *for*

CATARRH AND CATARRHAL DEAFNESS

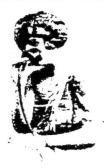

Great benefit is derived in cases of Catarrh by inhaling Ozone through the nostrils. Catarrh affects the nasal organs, and if neglected, afflicts the front cavities of the head, throat and tubes leading to the ears, also threatening the lungs. Renulife Violet Ray is especially useful in combating all Catarrhal conditions. Apply a mild current over the nose and forehead, then insert a small electrode No. 21 in the nostril, having the current turned off before doing so, then let the current pass from three to five minutes. Follow this by inhaling ozone. Almost immediate relief will be obtained.

"My wife suffered from Catarrhal Deafness. For years she has been left afflicted through Scarlet Fever, and while is now 42 years old, she never had the pleasure of knowing what her hearing meant. At Christmas time I brought home a Renulife Violet Ray Generator with Ozone attachment, and after four weeks of persistent treatment, my wife found that an accumulation of waste matter had been dislodged in her ear sufficient to have some part of it cling to the ear electrode. This was removed at the time that she took the electrode from her ear. At the same time a part of the congestion had dropped into her throat and from that moment she realized what it meant to have the use of her ears, as do those that have not afflictions.

"We have continuously used this equipment in our home since this accomplishment and we consider that it is the greatest asset for our health, it being so situated and connected so that every member of the family can avail themselves of the use of the machine without any inconvenience."

CONSTIPATION

Constipation is usually caused by sluggishness of the bowels; the nerves or muscles controlling their action are stimulated by applying Electrode No. 1 in contact with the abdomen for ten minutes daily. Renulife Violet Ray treatment restores the nerves and muscles to activity so that permanent recovery is effected. When laxatives are used, no permanent cure can be expected, but on the other hand, sluggishness is increased, and a chronic condition detrimental to health becomes permanent. Renulife Violet Ray is the best way to help nature in the treatment of constipation.

"Just a line to tell you I am getting along fine, and am free from constipation trouble. You can surely call me a renewed man."

Health - Strength - Beauty

COLD IN THE HEAD

Colds in the head are especially disagreeable, and relief can be found by applying No. 1 Electrode to the forehead, sides of nose and face in light contact for ten minutes twice daily, and inhaling ozone for ten minutes four times daily. Immediate relief may be expected.

DANDRUFF

Rake Comb Electrode No. 2 is especially designed for treatment of the scalp. Most troubles, such as falling hair, baldness, dandruff, are due to improper nourishment of the scalp cells. These cells starve for the life-giving oxygen which the blood should carry to them. Renulife Violet Ray restores the scalp to normalcy, stimulating the circulation of the blood, so that they again produce hair. At the same time the Renulife treatment destroys the bacterial and parasitic germs present which cause dandruff. The consistent use of Rake Comb Electrode No. 2 will end scalp troubles.

"I certainly enjoy the use of the Renulife I received from you, and I believe it will be of great benefit to me. Electrode No. 2 is a great dandruff loosener."

DEAFNESS

For Catarrhal Deafness, High Frequency current in connection with mechanical vibration yields remarkable results in 90% of the cases treated. Use insulated ear electrode No. 21 with a mild current for three to seven minutes daily. Marked improvement will result in practically every case.

"My hearing has improved wonderfully. In fact, my hearing in the left ear is almost normal now."

"I am still improving in hearing and general health conditions and can recommend the generator with confidence."

DYSPEPSIA

Renulife Violet Ray treatment, together with proper diet, brings relief from dyspepsia enabling the digestive organs to produce enough of the digestive juices to properly digest foods eaten. Use a strong current with Electrode No. 1 over the upper portion of the spine and over the stomach area. Take a treatment every day for ten minutes. Inhalations of ozone will be found very beneficial.

"We had a very severe case of indigestion in our family and I treated it with the Violet Ray, applying it twice daily, with the result that the patient was up and about the house within two days."

Renulife VIOLET RAY *for*

ECZEMA
(See also Acne and Skin Diseases)

In the treatment of Eczema, High Frequency current is invaluable. If the surface is dry, Electrode No. 1 may be used directly over the skin. If the area is moist, lay some thin gauze over the surface. Renulife treatment relieves itching, and good results are noted after the very first few treatments.

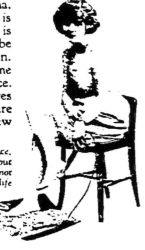

"Had weeping Eczema on my face, and have spent not hundreds but thousands of dollars, and still was not cured. After trying your Renulife Generator I noted good results after first few treatments and am now entirely well and my face perfectly smooth."

EARACHE

Earache is usually relieved by application of Electrode No. 21 inserted in the ear, using a moderate current. It is left there for three to ten minutes until the heat generated becomes uncomfortable. By this time the pain will have stopped, unless it is due to pressure back of the drum, in which case this treatment will not be effective.

Note: In all treatments of the ears be sure to have the ear electrode inserted before turning on the current and turn off before removing it.

ENLARGED PROSTATE (See Prostatic Diseases)

EYE DISEASES

Specialists find high frequency current invaluable in the treatment of eye diseases. In treating diseases of the eye, use the eye electrode in contact with the closed lid for not more than three minutes for each treatment. Treatments may be taken twice daily. Be sure to have the electrode in contact with the closed lid before turning the current on, and turn current off again before removing it. The revitalizing of the cells of the eye through Violet Ray is the reason for the improvement noted after taking these treatments. Electrode No. 16 is made to fit over one eye and double eye Electrode No. 17 is used for treating both eyes at the same time.

"I am having great success in the treatment of weak eyes."
"I have had the machine one week and am well pleased with it and my eyes are improving."

Health – Strength – Beauty

GOITER

Goiter is an enlargement of the thyroid gland. Many testimonials indicate splendid successes obtained by Renulife treatment of goiter. Electrode No. 1 or No. 4 is used to treat around and over the goiter.

"I have used the Renulife Violet Ray Generator in the treatment of my goiter with remarkable results. I used it twice daily. At the end of the first week my goiter began to decrease in size. At the end of three weeks it was entirely unnoticeable and I immediately began to feel better generally."

GRAY HAIR

Gray Hair, especially premature grayness, can be traced to lack of nourishment of the scalp cells. A woman who was being treated for baldness with High Frequency current, found that new hair coming in was natural color at the roots. Not only was baldness overcome but the natural black color was restored to the hair. Renulife treatment stimulates the circulation of the blood so that the proper nourishment is given the hair, and with proper nutrition the pigment which gives the hair color is restored. The treatment of gray hair calls for great persistence, but it meets with success.

GRIPPE (Influenza)

Inhalations of ozone are the quickest way to destroy the disease germs which attack the respiratory organs and cause Influenza and Grippe. Electrode No. 1 is also applied over the eyes, nose, spine and abdominal areas, and the small electrode No. 21 may be applied in each nostril. Grippe and Influenza are vicious diseases, leaving the patient in a debilitated condition. Renulife Violet Ray should be applied at the first sign of their appearance. The usefulness of Renulife in checking so many diseases at their very beginning—diseases which may become serious if no measures are taken to combat them—makes this instrument a household necessity. No home where health is valued can afford to be without one.

HAY FEVER

During an acute attack of Hay Fever a treatment every two or three hours with Electrode No. 21, which is placed in one nostril and then the other for

Renu*Life* VIOLET RAY *for*

from three to five minutes, followed by an inhalation of Ozone for ten minutes, brings decided relief. If a similar treatment is used daily for two weeks before the expected attack, it will frequently avert the attack of Hay Fever altogether or at least make it much milder.

"My husband, who is subject to hay fever suffered greatly with it after having flu. After just a few treatments of RenuLife Violet Ray he is almost cured."

WHERE HEADACHES OCCUR

Headaches at A or B are congestive or frontal. Eye trouble or frontal sinus or nasal disease may cause the ache at A. Such pain may also come from a disordered stomach. A-B, from constipation; C, anemia or bladder disease; D-E, from disorders of middle ear, or of throat, 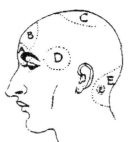 eyes or teeth; E, nervousness, spinal irritation or female trouble.

HEADACHES

Frontal or congestive headaches are almost instantly relieved by a treatment with Renulife Violet Ray. Violet Ray stimulates the circulation, enables the blood to throw off the poisons which are at the root of the disturbance, and improves the general physical condition. To relieve headaches caused by disturbances, such as disordered stomach, constipation, eyes or teeth, etc., as indicated above, it is necessary to eliminate the cause. (See sections of this booklet dealing with such disturbances.)

Headache and Nerves—"Received a Model M Generator and I am very pleased with it. My headache left me and my nerves are much quieter."

Headache Cured —"I bought a Model K which I used to treat a headache which I had for one year, and I am glad to say I was completely cured in two months."

Conscientious Statement —"I can conscientiously recommend the Violet Ray as being beneficial for the headache."

Prompt Relief —"I received my generator Model R just two days after I ordered it. I treated a headache and stopped it in three minutes."

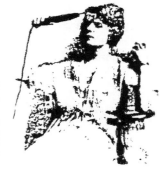

Health – Strength – Beauty

INSOMNIA

Sleeplessness, or Insomnia, is the result of overworked, tired nerves. Applications of the Renulife Violet Ray to all parts of the body and particularly the spine have a sedative, soothing effect. Nerves are quieted and in nearly all cases natural sleep quickly follows. Continued treatments build up and restore the entire nervous system to normal.

"Have found it of great value in relieving insomnia."

LUMBAGO

Lumbago is very successfully treated with Renulife Violet Ray. This is a disease which grips you in the small of the back. It is, in reality, rheumatism of the back. No matter how severe the pain, Renulife brings relief speedily, and normal conditions are completely restored in a few treatments at most.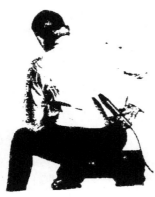

Apply through your clothing, to get the stimulating effect that brings circulation quickly to the part causing discomfort.

"I was down in bed with lumbago, unable to move unless I got help from someone. After one treatment of Renulife Violet Ray, I was able to get up the next morning. I have a machine at my home and would not be without it. I take great pleasure in recommending Violet Ray treatments to anyone who is afflicted with rheumatism or lumbago."

NERVOUS DISEASES

In treating the spinal column with Renulife Violet Ray current, the entire sympathetic nervous system is given a cellular massage which can only be obtained by this method of treatment. The most severe cases of nervous breakdown yield remarkably well to Renulife treatment. Ozone inhalations taken from five to ten minutes each day are also extremely beneficial.

"Renulife relieved me entirely of a serious case of nervous prostration, and I found it beneficial in various other ailments. I was a broken down person before its use, but am now entirely well and have used no other treatment than the generator."

NEURITIS

Neuritis is an inflamed condition of the nerves. The pain from it is similar to Rheumatism. The common form is Brachial Neuritis in the arm and shoulder. Violet Ray treatment over the painful area from three to five minutes twice a day quickly lessens the pain. With continued use of Renulife, the pain disappears altogether.

"I had neuritis in both my arms and sciatica in my left limb, and suffered so much I didn't know what a night's rest was. After taking fifteen treatments with Model M Generator, I sleep much better, and, whereas my limb was so painful I could only sit for about fifteen minutes, now I can sit as long as I please without discomfort."

NEURALGIA

Renulife Violet Ray is efficacious in the treatment of Neuralgia, which is caused by insufficient nutrition of the nerves. When the blood is below normal, the "starved nerve" cries out in pain. Renulife starts the blood circulating, feeds these nerves and restores them to normal health. Moreover, the oxygen contained in the blood is improved by Violet Ray, which improves nutrition. No one need suffer from Neuralgia or tortured nerves after obtaining a Renulife Health Generator.

"I purchased one of your Model "M" Generators about 5 weeks ago, primarily for neuralgia and nervousness. I have certainly found it all you claim. I would be glad to recommend this machine to any one."

PARALYSIS

Paralysis is not a disease, it is a symptom of certain forms of injury which cause the complete or partial loss of the motor function of the muscle fiber. Obstinate cases frequently require continued treatments for some time, but with patience, the cells are stimulated to life and the paralyzed muscles restored to use. Electrode No. 1 is applied over the paralyzed muscles and up and down the spine. Two treatments a day are advisable of from ten to fifteen minutes each.

"My affliction appeared to be extraordinary for a person to recover from as I have done. I had an attack of paralysis and my entire left side was afflicted. It also left me with very little desire for food, therefore my strength wasted quickly, but after the persistent application of your Violet Ray, I am gaining continually."

PROSTATIC DISEASES

Violet Ray has been found successful in the treatment of this distressing ailment common to so many men of middle age. Use Electrode No. 7 with medium to strong current, employing it through the rectum to reach prostate for an average of seven minutes. It may be used daily or twice a day in urgent cases. Be sure to turn the current off before electrode is inserted and again before removing it. The treatment as a rule should be taken under the advice of a competent physician.

"Early in July I bought a Model M Generator from your office, principally to treat myself for prostatic trouble and neuritis, and I want to tell you how much good it has been to me."

"The neuritis was eliminated within two weeks and has not bothered ~~some appearance.~~

"After doctoring for quite a while for what doctors said was prostatic trouble, I have used the generator as directed and can honestly say, I feel better in every way, and am not troubled as formerly, with that troublesome pain in the region of the prostate gland."

PYORRHEA

Violet Ray acts as a tonic to the spongy tissue of pyorrhea-infected gums. Loosened teeth are tightened and bleeding of the gums stopped. Use Electrode No. 44 in the treatment directly in contact with the gums.

RHEUMATISM (See Lumbago)

High frequency currents are of exceptional value in muscular and chronic articular rheumatism. In the acute articular form it is of comparatively little value. Renulife Violet Ray treatment reduces the uric acid in the system and relieves inflammation and pain.

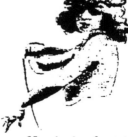

Treatments should be taken every day and should cover the whole affected area. Hundreds of testimonials indicate the effectiveness of Renulife in treating rheumatism.

"I want to tell you what Renulife Violet Ray has done for me. It has put me on my feet after being a cripple for 14 years. At times I could not walk at all. I had rheumatism from my hips down to my feet. Everyone is surprised how good I can walk now—thanks to the Renulife Generator."

RenuLife VIOLET RAY *for Health - Strength - Beauty*

KEEP WELL AT HOME

Renulife Violet Ray Generator Most Efficient. Compact. Durable. Low Priced

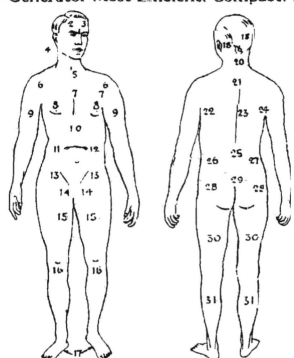

The hundreds of testimonials we are receiving from satisfied users prove conclusively that we have achieved our aim. that of placing within the reach of every one the means of renewing or restoring the HEALTH to normal. To date the greatest drawback has been the enormous cost of the instruments. making treatments possible only for those who could afford to spend a small fortune in renewing their HEALTH. Hospitals and specialists have used large instruments for years, being forced to charge large payments for their treatments. In placing our generators on the market, we have placed the most efficient health builder known to science at a price that is within the reach of every one.

In this booklet we touch briefly on some of the uses of Renulife Generators. Directions for applying treatment for various ailments listed are given in detail in the treatment chart, and directions for use, accompanying each generator.

ABBREVIATED TREATMENT CHART. USING ELECTRODE No. 1

Rheumatism: Treat area of pain through thin layer of clothing. also apply to 11-12, 26-27.

Headache: Apply to 2, 3, 1, 20, 21, 23, 11-12.

Insomnia: Apply to 11-12. 26-27. down spine from nape of neck to 25. also apply to bottom of feet 17.

Neuralgia of the Face: Apply to cheeks, front of ear, and cords of neck.

Indigestion: Treat 12-11. 10, 20, 23-25.

Constipation: Treat 13-13, 14-14. 12-11.

Nervousness: Treat area at 19, also up and down spine from 19 to 29. Treat 18-18, also treat abdominal region 13, 14, 12, 11, also upper arms and shoulders 6-9, also lower limbs, 31, 17.

Deafness: Treat all around back and front of ear, also internal ear with electrode No. 21.

Dandruff, Falling Hair, Gray Hair, and Scalp Ailments : Electrode No. 1 may be used. but rake comb electrode No. 2 preferred. Cover entire scalp at least once a day, eight-minute treatments.

Complexion: In addition to applying to face and neck, treat for improved digestion in area 12-11.

To Strengthen Lungs and Develop Chest: Thoroughly cover area 5-8, 5-7, also area 21-22, 21-24, holding up chest and breathing deeply during treatment; ozone inhalation from ozone generator is very desirable.

ONE FULL YEAR'S GUARANTEE ACCOMPANIES EVERY RENULIFE.

Renulife VIOLET RAY for

Health — Strength — Beauty

SCIATICA

Hundreds of testimonials from users prove that Sciatica is successfully treated with Renulife Violet Ray. Apply No. 1 Electrode along the course of the nerve and over the lower part of the spine. The irritated nerves are quickly soothed, pain disappears.

"I had a steady ache in my hip and my foot, ankles and calf were swollen badly. I had had nothing but slippers on all summer, but in the last two weeks by using the Renulife generator twice a day, the ache in my hip has practically left me and I can now jump curbstones, get on and off trolley cars."

SKIN DISEASES
(See Also Acne and Eczema)

Electrode No. 1 is employed over the area affected, with usually a medium strength current for about five to eight minutes daily.

"I had been subjected to pimples for almost five years and had tried everything, vibrators and all, but with no results. I have just used your generator one week, as I was out of the city when it came. Today my face is as clear as anyone could ever wish for."

SORE THROAT, HOARSENESS, TONSILITIS

All cases of hoarseness, loss of voice, throat infections caused by congestion, are successfully treated by applying Electrodes No. 1 and No. 4 from five to ten minutes over the front and sides of the throat. Ozone inhalations are also of distinct benefit. Actors, speakers and singers find Violet Ray treatment of great benefit. Congestion and inflammation are rapidly relieved and the nervous mechanism of the vocal organs toned up with amazing quickness.

"Using one of your Renulife Violet Ray generators for a short time has assisted wonderfully in relieving my throat before singing."

SPRAINS

Use Electrode No. 1 in direct contact with the surface. For old sprains, use sufficient spark to produce marked reddening of the skin.

"After I sprained my ankle, I limped around for about a week with a cane, and it seemed to get no better. Finally, I went over and got my Renulife Violet Ray machine from some friends to whom I had loaned it, and to my surprise, I obtained immediate relief upon using it. I used it steadily until my ankle was completely cured."

WRY NECK (Torticollis)

Wry Neck or stiff neck in a sub-acute form is relieved by a treatment with Electrode No. 1 in back of the ears and down the back and sides of the neck.

"For eight years I was afflicted with a stiff, sore neck. After taking three Renulife treatments, to my great surprise, I felt some relief, and after eight treatments I was entirely cured and could turn my head and twist my neck without the least pain."

TREATING AT NERVE CENTERS

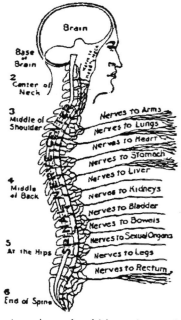

In the spine are centered nerves radiating to every part of the body. This is roughly shown in the accompanying illustration.

Chiropractors treat entirely upon the spine to relieve ailments in any part of the body. We have found also that Violet Ray treatments on the spine are very beneficial in addition to the regular local treatments; for instance, if indigestion is present, in addition to the direct treatment of the stomach region, there should be a thorough going over the middle back at the point marked 4 on the accompanying chart, or if headache is to be treated, as well as going over the forehead or the place where the pain is apparent, treatment should be taken at the base of the skull just where the nerves to the head and neck connect with the spine. This treatment brings nutrition and nourishment to the nerves and helps them to alleviate the trouble. In like manner the proper nerve center should be treated for any ailment, in addition to the local application. This indirect (nerve center) application will prove of much benefit in treating organic disorders.

In all nervous troubles, including nervous breakdown, neurasthenia, insomnia, nervous debility, neuritis, etc., and also for building up the body generally, treatment should be taken over the entire length of the spine. Where a quieting or sedative effect is desired, treatment should be in direct contact with the body with a medium current; where a stimulating current is desired, or where it is necessary to eliminate pain, sparks should be applied or treatment taken through medium thick clothing with a medium strength current.

RenuLife VIOLET RAY *for*

RENULIFE UNEQUALLED FOR BEAUTY CULTURE

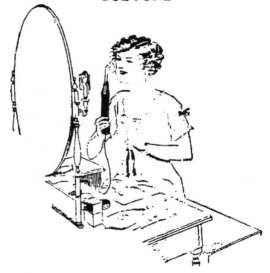

All beauty parlors today have adopted the Violet Ray as essential equipment. Our Renulife Violet Ray Generators designed for self treatments, virtually bring to your home all the advantages of the modern beauty shop. In fact, you are enabled to effect even more gratifying results than are possible through an occasional treatment at the hands of an expert, because daily you may make use of this wonderful agency which works with Nature to refresh and restore.

Its cosmetic value is particularly great, as it delivers its vibrating impulses into the tissues at a rate of frequency infinitely higher than any mechanical vibrator, and without stretching and "sagging" the skin or scalp. Parasitic bacteria that destroy the hair follicles and produce disfiguring eruptions are destroyed and eliminated while dormant nerve cells are galvanized into normal functioning.

FOR SKIN AND COMPLEXION

The Violet Ray treatment is delightfully pleasant, and is the most effective method ever discovered to retain a youthful appearance and to gain beauty. It will remove blemishes, warts, moles, wrinkles, crows feet, pouches under the eyes, blackheads and sagging lines of the face and chin. A single treatment will convince you that it is a crime against yourself to be without a Renulife Generator when all marks and lines can be so quickly removed.

Health — Strength — Beauty

Besides the direct facial treatment with surface electrode, which treatment you can readily give yourself, you will find it very beneficial to hold in your hand the general electrode, or preferably the metal electrode, while another person massages your face with the hands. This draws the stimulating sparks to the surface thus massaged.

FACIAL MASSAGE

Cleanse the face thoroughly with cleansing cream. Then lightly run Electrode No. 1 over the skin to invigorate it and bring out healthy natural color. This treatment clears up muddiness, eliminates pimples and blackheads. Finish by cleansing with Witch Hazel or toilet water, and apply powder or rouge as desired. A daily Renulife Treatment will make you look years younger.

FILLS OUT AND DEVELOPS

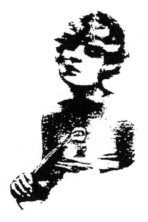

The Violet Ray is applied through the surface electrode as a massage. When the face, chin, neck, and bust are treated with the Violet Ray, the blood is brought to the surface, the soft muscles are gently massaged, the lines fill out, the wrinkles disappear, and the bloom of health is renewed.

RELIEVING FATIGUE

Proper rest is essential to beauty and health. During sleep the fatigue poisons and waste tissue are removed from the blood, and the body is refreshed and invigorated. Renulife Violet Ray in a few minutes' time supplies the oxygen to the blood that hours of sleep produce. Massage the back of the neck, the forehead and the spine with Electrode No. 1.

OZONE CREATED BY RENULIFE VIOLET RAY

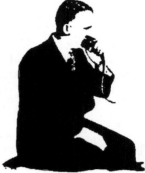

Ozone is simply a concentrated form of oxygen. Without oxygen we cannot live. When we breathe we fill the lungs full of air. The oxygen in the air passes through the walls of the lungs, purifying the blood, which is flowing through the walls of the lungs and which comes there from every part of the body to be purified.

It is the lack of pure air to purify our blood that causes us to be overcome with disease. Being cooped up in an office or factory all day long is responsible for many of our diseases and particularly diseases of the respiratory organs.

WHAT AUTHORITIES SAY

"Germs are destroyed by Ozone, and it has been shown capable of so thoroughly disinfecting sewage that the filtered water was pronounced suitable for drinking purposes."

"In Chlorosis and Anemia, Ozone inhalations are exceedingly valuable from a therapeutic standpoint, and give better and prompter results than any other forms of medication."

"Ozone is the remedy par excellence for Whooping Cough."

RENULIFE OZONE GENERATORS

The Renulife Ozone Generators deliver Ozone in large quantities for inhalation purposes. The Ozone penetrates every cell in the lungs, purifying the blood, destroying disease germs and soothing the inflamed tissues. For Asthma, Catarrh, Hay Fever, Coughs, Colds, Bronchitis, Tuberculosis, etc., Ozone treatments are particularly beneficial.

Our Ozone inhaler attachment No. 25 is designed to fit the handle of any Renulife Generator.

High Frequency Current conducted through this attachment creates Ozone in quantities, confines it and filters through Pine Needle Oil so that one may inhale it with maximum benefits.

Pine Needle Oil, a mixture of oil of Eucalyptus and oil of Pine Needles, has a soothing effect on the membranes and reduces oxides of nitrogen back to the original form of nitrogen and oxygen.

This glass Ozone Generator No. 25, fits handle of all Renulife models, furnishes Ozone for inhaling. Price **$9.50**

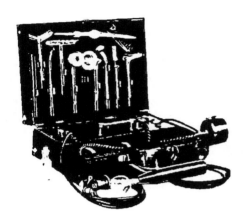

Model "R"

The most complete portable High Frequency Violet Ray Generator manufactured; for both professional and home use; delivers two qualities of High Frequency current and includes highly efficient built-in Ozone Generator with inhaling mask. A simple selective switch brings into use Ozone Inhaler or High Frequency (Violet Ray) treatment with strong, penetrating current for external treatment or exceedingly smooth, soothing current for internal treatment. Beautifully finished in black seal grain leatherette with extra heavy nickel corners, lock and carrying handle. Consumes approximately 50 watts of electricity. Case is dust-proof and has rich purple velvet lining; size of case 14¾ x 10½ x 5½ inches. Includes two Electrodes No. 1, one No. 2 Rake Comb, one No. 3 Saturator, one No. 4 External Throat, one No. 6 Internal Throat, one No. 8 Rectal, one No. 14 Fulguration, one No. 15 Spinal, one No. 16 Single Eye, one No. 18 Condenser Electrode and one bottle of Pine Needle Oil for Ozone Generator.

Model "R" is recommended for the treatment of deep-seated or chronic afflictions, such as rheumatism, lumbago, sciatica and neuritis.

Price **$75.00**

RenuLife VIOLET RAY *for*

Health - Strength - Beauty

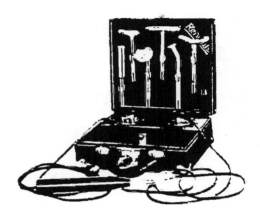

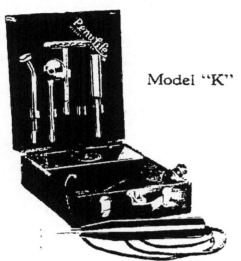

Model "K"

Model "M"

A most substantial all-round outfit for general use: built in self-contained carrying case, size 12 x 10½ x 4¼ inches, handsomely finished in black seal grain leatherette with heavy nickel corners and lock; highly polished mahogany finish top plate, dust-proof case lined with rich purple velvet. Consumes approximately 38 watts of electricity. Three-way switch allows operator to select current for internal or external use or shut instrument off entirely; includes two General Body Electrodes; one No. 2 Rake Comb; one No. 3 Saturator; one No. 4 External Throat; one No. 15 Spinal, and one No. 16 Single Eye Electrode.

Any Renulife instrument can be supplied to operate on 32, 110, 220 or any other voltage between these limits, direct or alternating current. An instrument will operate only on the voltage for which designed. Unless otherwise ordered, the 110 volt outfit is supplied. No Extra Charge for Voltage Varying from 110.

Model "M" generates a powerful high frequency current which makes it ideal to use in the treatment of rheumatism, lumbago, sciatica, neuritis and other deep-seated or chronic ailments.

Price. $45.00

A very popular outfit for all-around use: built in self-contained carrying case; compact and efficient; top plate beautiful mahogany finish; case solid wood covered with seal grain leatherette; purple velvet lined. Adjustment of current by knob on top plate; consumes approximately 30 watts of electricity. Size of case 9 x 10 x 4 inches. Two General Surface Electrodes, one No. 2 Rake Comb, one No. 3 Saturator and one No. 16 Single Eye Electrode included. Price $30.00

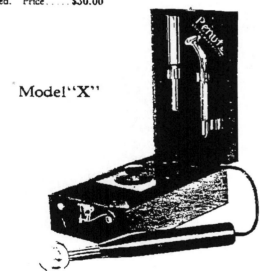

Model "X"

An exceptionally attractive Generator made to sell at low price, without sacrificing therapeutic value and durability. Case covered with seal grain leatherette and lined with purple velvet; top plate mahogany finished; adjustment of current by knob on top plate. Size of case 10½ x 6½ x 3¾ inches. Consumes approximately 11 watts of electricity. Complete as shown. Includes General Body Electrode No. 1; Saturator Electrode No. 3 and Single Eye Electrode No. 16. Price. $22.50

Renulife VIOLET RAY for

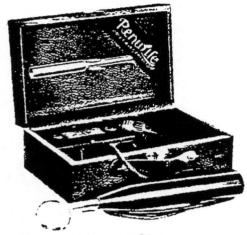

Model "H"

This efficient Cabinet Generator offers the greatest possible value for the amount invested. The Generator is built in a carrying case covered with seal grain leatherette. Adjustment knob to control strength of current. Consumes approximately 15 watts of electricity. A General Body Electrode No. 1 and a Saturator Electrode No. 3 included.
Price.................................$12.50

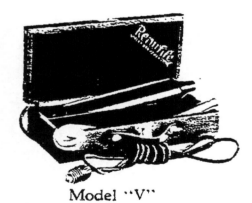

Model "V"

This all-in-handle (one-piece) instrument offers the greatest efficiency possible in this type of Generator. Size of instrument 10½ inches long by 2 inches diameter; 7 foot connector cord. Equipment includes the carrying case substantially built: leatherette covered, satin lined: size 11¼ x 5¼ x 2⅞ inches. A general body Electrode No. 1, and a Saturator Electrode No. 3 included. Consumes approximately 15 watts of electricity. Price . $12.50

Health – Strength – Beauty

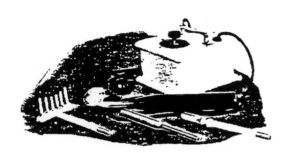

Beauty Parlor Model "G"

This instrument has been especially designed for Beauty Parlor and Barber Shop use. It is made to withstand continued use and is equipped with coils, etc., to deliver the current best adapted for hair, scalp, massage and facial treatments.

The case is beautifully finished in white enamel with all metal parts nickeled. An extra length of connector cord facilitates the movements of the operator in giving treatments. Size 7¼ x 5½ x 3¾ inches.

This handsome outfit complete with General Surface Electrode No. 1, Rake Comb Scalp Electrode No. 2, Metal Saturator Electrode No. 3 for indirect massage and Fulguration Electrode No. 14.
Price.................................$27.50

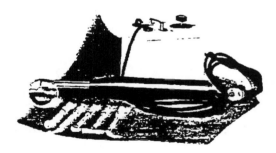

Model "D"

Dental model in white enamel finish. High Frequency current of a character best suited for dental work. Electrodes as shown included.
Price $32.50

RenuLife VIOLET RAY *for*

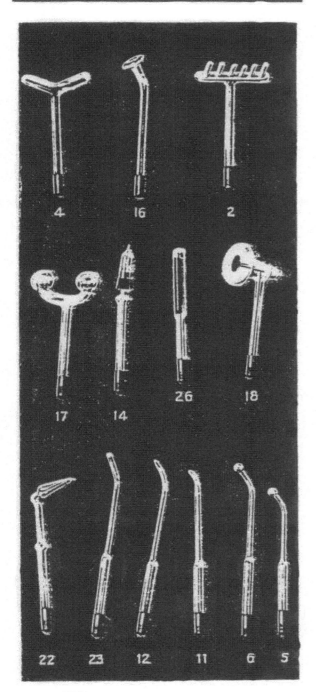

See page 28 for description of electrodes and prices

Health-Strength-Beauty

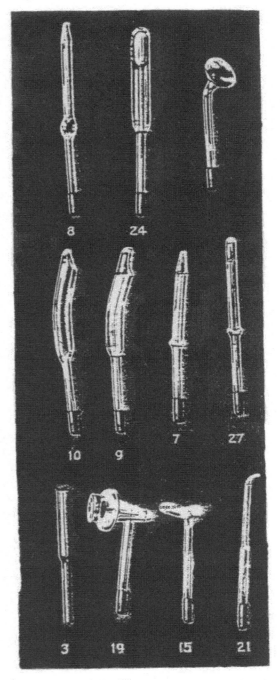

See page 28 for description of electrodes and prices

CHAPTER VI

Testimonials on the Use of the Violet Ray

"I have found the Violet Ray good for something other than the cataract protocol. I am 78 and have joined other seniors in having trouble with bruises on my hands and forearms…resulting from very slight knocks. The doctors seem to feel nothing can be done about it. They say I should have used more sun lotion in the past.

"The Violet Ray will break up these bruises and they will start diminishing in a day or two. It used to take a week to 10 days for them to diminish. I assume the Violet Ray stimulates the circulation and that is what begins reducing the bruise." *Case #112650 D.C., Texas*

"I love my VR, I haven't had a sinus headache in a long time and my skin is improving." *Case #170413, L.S., AZ*

"I had hit my knee against something right in an area where there had been surgery a few years earlier. It was very painful and bruised quickly, and made walking painful. I was worried I had hurt something inside. The Violet Ray was recommended to help with the bruising, and even though I knew there were plates and screws within (titanium maybe?), I used the VR for just a few minutes. Within 12 hours the knee felt great again and I was able to go back to exercising without pain. The bruising disappeared as well." *Case #159165, L.N., PA*

"I once cured a lady of CFS (Chronic Fatigue Syndrome) with one treatment of the Violet Ray over her spine." *Case #5, T.J., VA*

"Two months of twice daily use with the Violet Ray have yielded the following results;
"My back has re-adjusted— rib ends and vertebrae gently "pop" back into place. And no more

pain from a whiplash neck injury. Despite weekly chiropractic appointments, one thoracic rib head had been "out" for an entire year. I'm thrilled to be able to fire my chiropractor!

"Within seconds it relaxes my entire system. No more costly cranial osteopathy at $200 a pop. For this benefit alone, the Violet Ray has more than paid for itself.

"It has provided the "spark" I have been missing in my system. It lifted my spirits and actually makes me happy. I can't wait to use it each day.

"When my calves cramped up one night causing restless legs syndrome so bad I couldn't get to sleep, I got up and applied the Violet Ray. It alleviated the cramp in a few minutes of use.

"It has completely cleared my facial acne, including cystic acne which is so hard to eliminate. My skin is tighter too, although it relaxes the tight facial muscles. My sister in law, who is an esthetician, swears by this device for this purpose and says she routinely waves brides from embarrassing breakouts on their big days.

"My doctor recommended ozone treatments to me but I was never able to handle the smell. In contrast, the ozone generated by the Violet Ray is mild and refreshing and I enjoy it.

"I have been treating Lyme Disease for the past 3 years (misdiagnosed with chronic fatigue and fibromyalgia for 10 years) and have spent hundreds of thousands of dollars on treatments, devices, and doctors trying to get well. After failed antibiotic treatment, I found the success with the Gerson Protocol (coffee enemas and juicing), fife machine, parasite cleansing, metal detoxing, and infra-red sauna sessions. However, nothing has given me results as quickly as the Violet Ray. One of the hallmarks of Lyme is thickening of the blood and stiffening joints where the organism lives. It seems to me that the Violet Ray alleviates both conditions, thus allowing the body to heal itself.

"Incidentally, I am a research biologist who could not have been more skeptical about such devices when I first got sick. Now I tell everyone about it, especially people with chronic diseases. I believe that it provides the missing link to complete healing." *Case #179288, A.F., NM*

"A thank you for the help with the Violet Ray. I am grateful for the demonstration which made it very comfortable for me to use it here at home.

"My chiropractor used the Violet Ray on my spine last week for 10 min. As the result, I had almost no back pain for 2 days.

"I will be getting a Violet Ray treatment from him once a week for four weeks and then decide where to go from there.

"Meanwhile, I treat my own hands and feet for pain, stiffness, and also some numbness in the right foot because of years of ill-fitting shoes and pressure on a tailor's bunion." *Case #229038, J.R., PA*

"I recently attended the Dr. Bruce Baar/Cayce seminar in St. Pete. Dr. Baar was very knowledgeable and a good presenter. I ordered the Violet Ray machine – it's turning my life around."   *C. R., FL*

"I used the Violet Ray with just the bulb electrode that comes with it on my scalp last night. I think I got the best night's sleep ever after that."   *Case #225951, H.H., MO*

"I thought you would like to know this. I tried using the Violet Ray to treat my sister for varicose veins in her leg. They were severe and discolored. After daily treatments for three weeks the veins were shrinking. We were all thrilled."   *Case #79057, N.Q., NJ*

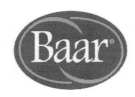

OTHER TITLES BY BRUCE BAAR, MS, ND

Carbondex, Carbon Ash & Animated Ash Reference Manual
Castor Oil Pack Therapy
Electrical Immune Therapy and Multiple Sclerosis
Experience The Radiac
Parkinson's Report
Scleroderma Report

VIDEO TITLES BY BAAR PRODUCTS, INC.

Baar® Wet Cell Instructional DVD

Baar Products, Inc.
PO Box 60
Downingtown, PA 19335 USA
610-873-4591
www.baar.com

ISBN: 978-1539586302
THIRD EDITION

Made in the USA
Columbia, SC
05 May 2021